Patient Testimonials

As I approached middle age, severe headaches became a real problem for me. By following Dr. Walsh's suggestions, I've been able to decrease the number of headaches and completely control the few I continue to have.

—C.N.A.

Headaches and other allergy-related symptoms are often aggravated, or even caused, by items in our homes or offices that are designed to improve our lives. It is important to focus on home and office designs that enhance the comfort of the allergy-sensitive person.

—G.L.F.

Five years ago, severe headaches that kept me in bed and barely functional for days at a time were fairly routine. Since changing my diet, adjusting my environment, getting regular allergy shots, and knowing what preventive medications to take, and when, those headaches are history!

—M.P.

From a fellow physician . . .

As a medical doctor, I find it necessary to be well educated and current in the diagnosis and treatment of eczema, hay fever, and asthma, for allergic patients are common in one's practice. As the father of a young son with migraine headaches, I was stimulated to be constantly acquiring knowledge about headaches.

However, in more than forty-five years of study in medical school, internship, residency, postgraduate courses at Harvard, yearly medical refresher projects, Audio-Digest tapes, and innumerable medical journals, never once did any lecturer or author in allergy or in neurology ever hint at a possible connection between foods and airborne antigens such as dust mites, molds, and pollen and some recurring headaches.

In recent years, patients began to tell me of Dr. Walsh's success in helping them control the headaches they had endured for several years. His book on the relationships between some repetitive headaches and allergy is most enlightening and welcome. Although Dr. Walsh's writing style is anecdotal rather than statistical and is aimed at the layperson, I strongly encourage every general practitioner, pediatrician, internist, and neurologist to read this publication. Integration of his thoughts into their therapeutic programs will benefit many patients with distressing, recurrent headaches.

—Albert E. Miller, M.D.

Treating Sinus, Migraine, and Cluster Headaches, My Way

*An Allergist's Approach to
Headache Treatment*

Treating Sinus, Migraine, and Cluster Headaches, My Way

An Allergist's Approach to Headache Treatment

William E. Walsh, M.D.

ACA Publications, Inc.
St. Paul, Minnesota

Designed and Composed by Barbara Field

ACA Publications, Inc.
1690 University Avenue West, Suite 450
St. Paul, Minnesota 55104

Printed in the United States of America

Contents

Preface

"Dr. Walsh, if I had known that allergy caused my headaches, I would have come to you for treatment years ago."

How frequently patients express this sentiment, and how often in almost these exact words. Patients who, when they first come to my office, suffer from headaches that make their heads throb with unrelenting pressure or pound with excruciating pain—headaches that torment them during the day and interrupt their sleep at night.

They need not suffer such pain. Their sinus, migraine, and cluster headaches often arise from a malfunction of the immune system, a malfunction called allergy. Correcting this malfunction reverses many of the illnesses of allergy, of which headache is one of the most prominent.

Modern medicine gives allergists powerful tools to do this. For years I have used these tools, and, although I know their effectiveness, I am still delighted at their ability to soothe persistent and painful headaches. Nothing gives me more pleasure than to see my patients' smiles when they tell me how much better they feel.

Although I am gratified by how effective allergy treatment is in providing pain relief, I can't help wondering if my nurses and I could be even more effective. I often ask myself: *Is there a better way to instruct our patients? Is there a way to reach more people with our message?*

We teach those who come to our office about the conditions in their homes, schools, and workplaces that cause their headaches and tell them how to correct these conditions. We also identify the foods and beverages that cause headaches and provide a diet plan that replaces them with less troublesome foods and beverages. But, in the short time they spend in our office, and with the many distractions that may divert their attention, do they receive enough instruction? Is there a better way to teach them about allergy?

I discovered there is. For a number of years, I published a newsletter covering many topics related to allergy, and my patients told me how much they appreciated getting the information and how well they understood what they read. I realized that if I wrote a book about allergy-related illnesses, I could use their ability for self-instruction to help them better understand and treat their own headaches.

This treatment requires changes in both the diet and the environment, and since each of these areas requires detailed instructions, I knew I could not adequately cover both in one book. I decided to tackle the diet first. I wrote and published *Treating Food Allergy, My Way,* a book that describes the foods that cause chronic allergic symptoms, including headaches. As I had hoped, when my patients read the book, their understanding of food allergy increased and they found it much easier to avoid the offending foods and beverages.

To help defray the costs of publishing the book, I agreed to make it available in bookstores. Its reception was far greater than I had anticipated. So many people purchased it that the original printing, which should have lasted three to five years, was almost gone within a year. Realizing that the book would have to be reprinted, I decided to update and expand it to make it more informative, and the revised edition is now available.

With that task completed, I decided it was time to look specifically at one chronic illness—headaches—and describe a successful approach to overcoming this painful disorder. We will start by learning about the immune system to help in understanding how it gives rise to allergy and how allergy causes headaches. The first part of the book is devoted to this explanation.

Next, we will explore how head pain is precipitated by problems in the environment. Unless these problems are understood and eliminated, the causes of allergic headaches will continue to be an enigma and treatment will continue to be frustrating. This need not be so. These problems are not only understandable, they can be changed, and the results of making such changes are gratifying.

Finally we will look at the tools available for treating allergy—the all-important patient history, the skin test, and allergy injections. They allow the allergist to approach the treatment of headaches with great confidence that if his patients can understand and cooperate in modifying the dietary and environmental factors that cause their headaches, their pain can be alleviated.

As the title of the book suggests, the methods we will examine are ones my nurses and I have developed over many years of treating our patients. These methods need not be confined to our office. We use no unusual or revolutionary tests or treatments. We only combine those that have been available for years into a systematic approach to diagnosis and management that has proven successful in reducing and ultimately eliminating the pain endured by many allergy sufferers.

The principles we use can be applied by pediatricians, internists, and family doctors, and certainly by other allergists, and I hope they will do so. The millions who suffer sinus, migraine, and cluster headaches need the relief our methods provide. In the meantime, may this book help our patients to better understanding and help those who are not our patients to confront and subdue the cruel headaches that plague them.

Acknowledgments

This book describes a successful method for treating allergic headaches, a method I did not discover by myself. Rather, my patients taught it to me. In sharing their thoughts about the causes of their headaches, they guided me in discarding ineffective treatments and in retaining those that are worthwhile. To my patients, a heartfelt thank you.

My thanks also to those noble women and men who serve in the front line of medical care—the family doctors, pediatricians, and internists. Most of the patients I treat were referred to me by these doctors. Without their support, my practice would not exist, and this method of treating headaches would never have evolved.

Just as the help of my patients was essential in developing this treatment, so was the assistance of the nurses who serve with me. Each is a registered nurse with many years of experience in treating the allergic patient. Their help is essential in initial evaluation and diagnosis, in making environmental and dietary recommendations, and in providing continuing injection treatment. A sincere thank you to Shirley Hess, Arleen Nietz, Corinne Peterson, and Jan Ryan.

I also want to acknowledge the contributions of Peter Bergh and Doctors Al Heimel and Al Miller, whose comments helped shape this manuscript, and those of Barbara Field,

whose hard work and editorial skill smoothed many awkward sentences and illuminated many murky passages.

Finally, many others have contributed to this method of
treatment and to this book. To all of you, my deepest grati-
tude.

WILLIAM E. WALSH   APRIL 1993

The case histories described in this book are representative of many conversations with patients who have similar illnesses and food allergies. They are included to help the reader understand the allergic headache and its treatment. Although the essence of each case history is preserved, the names, occupations, and certain facts have been changed to prevent recognition of the patients and protect their privacy.

Part I
Allergy and Headaches

Allergy Causes Headaches?

You might think that after years of treating headaches, there would be no surprises for me. But that is not the case. I continue to be amazed that so many people, including doctors, are unaware that allergy causes headaches.

This lack of awareness is very apparent in the new patients we see. They come to our office for treatment of hives, or asthma, or diarrhea, or any of the many illnesses brought on by the diet and environment. Many also have headaches, but few realize that allergy causes not only their hives, asthma, and diarrhea but also their headaches. Their faces reflect their surprise when I question them about their head pain, a problem they never thought would concern an allergist. They often ask, "Allergies don't cause headaches, do they?"

Yes, allergy does cause headaches, and the best evidence of that comes from the patients who make up my practice. Among these allergic patients, headaches strike often and painfully. Allergy frequently causes headaches.

I deeply regret this lack of awareness about allergy-related headaches among doctors and patients. Not knowing about allergy's power to cause pain is as much a barrier to receiving helpful medical care as is the lack of a doctor to administer this care. What is the difference between patients who suffer because they lack medical care and patients who suffer because they are unaware that allergy causes their headaches? To me, there is no difference.

Although I can't solve the problems brought on by lack of access to medical care, I can spread the word that allergy causes headaches. With this knowledge, headache sufferers can receive the appropriate treatment to fight their miserable head pains.

You are most likely reading this book because you or someone close to you has frequent headaches and you want the answers to some or all of the following questions. Where do the headaches come from? Why do I or my loved one get headaches? How do I find out if my headaches are caused by allergy? Why do I feel so awful when I have a headache?

I hope to provide answers to these questions. However, just as a teacher needs to teach her class to count to ten before she can teach them to add and subtract, I need to give you a basic explanation of the immune system before I can answer your questions. Once you learn about this vitally important system and the key role is plays in sprouting the seeds of allergy, the answers to these questions will become apparent.

Let's begin our journey to understanding the symptoms and causes of allergy by looking at the amazing immune system.

The Immune System

Your body is made up of many systems that are essential to life. Without them you would die. You are probably familiar with many of them, such as your breathing system—the airways and lungs—and your circulatory system—the heart and blood vessels. But there is another, less familiar system at work inside your body that is equally as necessary to life. Although the signs that it is functioning aren't as apparent as your beating heart or your regular breathing, your immune system is working hard at all times, quietly killing germs. Without it you would quickly die of massive infection from the germs that surround you in the air, live in your food, and grow and multiply on your skin.

Your immune system is like your own personal army—fighting germs the way our armed forces fight the enemies of our country. They are even organized in a similar way. Each has a certain number of scouts to identify the enemy and a main body of troops to do the actual fighting. However, although there are similarities between your immune system and a regular army, there are also differences. The regular army fights on land, but your immune army fights its battles in the salty fluid that flows through your blood vessels.

Long ago our primitive ancestors left the safety of the salty oceans for dry land, but they never entirely left the sea behind. They took it with them in the bloodstream, where the immune army swims. (One of the reasons our ancestors were able to leave the ocean and walk the land is that they developed skin to prevent dehydration. Our skin still serves this water-conserving function today, proving it is a vital organ and more than just a surface on which to grow whiskers, apply cosmetics, and slap mosquitoes.)

The bloodstream flows through the blood vessels to every part of our bodies. It penetrates the liver, kidneys, lungs, heart, and muscles. It communicates with the fluid that surrounds and cushions these organs. Because it penetrates every inch of us, and because it carries our army of germ killers with it, the immune system can reach any area of the body.

Unfortunately, the same bloodstream that carries the immune system also carries the germs that invade and infect us. The battle between the immune army and the invading germs takes place in this soggy environment of the bloodstream and in the fluid surrounding our organs. To understand how this battle is waged, we must delve further into the salty water that carries both immunity and germs throughout the body.

The Scouts

In our immune army, the scouts are called *antigen-presenting cells* (an antigen is a tiny bit of matter, such as a piece of an infecting germ, found somewhere in the body where it does not belong). The antigen-presenting cell searches endlessly through the bloodstream, tirelessly looking for any bits of unfamiliar material (antigen) that signal an invasion by infecting germs. Its eternal vigilance pays off when it come across a piece of flu virus floating in the blood, an enemy fully capable of destroying the body if it is not stopped and destroyed.

But the antigen-presenting cell can't destroy the millions of invading flu viruses. It only pauses long enough to grab the piece of flu virus—like a scout taking a prisoner for interrogation—and rapidly swims off to warn the main army of the immune system that flu viruses are invading.

The Lymphocytes

The foot soldiers of the immune system are the *lymphocytes.* Their task is to destroy the invading germs and stem the tide of infection. And just like a human army, in which each soldier is trained to do a specific job, the lymphocytes are also highly specialized. Only a limited number are specifically programmed to fight a particular attacking germ. To defeat the invading flu viruses, the antigen-presenting cell must find those few flu-fighting lymphocytes.

Hanging onto its piece of flu virus, the antigen presenting cell swims from lymphocyte to lymphocyte until it finds one capable of fighting the flu. It presents the offending piece to this lymphocyte, called a *T lymphocyte,* a hunter–killer cell that has been slumbering quietly until that moment. Like a sleeping soldier is roused by the morning bugle call, the T lymphocyte awakens to the horrifying realization that its host's bloodstream has been invaded by millions of flu germs. Unless it stops them, the body will die.

But the awakened lymphocyte faces a frightening problem. It can only find a few soldier–lymphocytes that are specially trained in fighting flu viruses to join the battle, but the flu invasion is massive. It needs help and it needs it fast.

To recruit this help, the T lymphocyte rapidly divides itself into two cells, then those two cells divide into four, the four divide into eight, and so on, until thousands of identical flu-killing lymphocytes are charging through the bloodstream, attacking every flu virus they find. But even this impressive force of lymphocytes cannot defeat the entire flu virus invasion. They face an obstacle that, by themselves, they cannot overcome.

The problem is their size. The blood vessels in which the T lymphocytes swim are connected in an unbroken series of tubes suspended in the body's fluid. The lymphocytes swim through these tubes like enormous whales in an endless underwater tunnel, far too large to escape through the minute openings in the sides of the blood vessels.

Unfortunately, the blood vessel walls are no barrier for the tiny flu viruses. They escape through the minute holes, invading the body fluid and spreading an epidemic of flu into each watery crevice of the body, safe from the killing power of the whale–lymphocytes trapped in the blood vessels. To save the body from this death-dealing infection, the lymphocytes must also break free of the confining vessels to attack the flu virus.

Realizing that they need to escape, the lymphocytes release chemicals that flow through the bloodstream until they seek out and awaken another sleeping cell, a different type of lymphocyte called a *B lymphocyte*.

This B lymphocyte is like a factory ship with all its machinery shut down. It drifts lazily through the blood vessels until it is awakened by the call for help from the T lymphocyte. Firing up its boilers, switching on its machines, and activating its production lines, the B lymphocyte begins to flood the bloodstream with its products. These products are called *antibodies*.

The Antibodies

Antibodies are proteins made by the B lymphocytes. To understand how they work, visualize them as built like the fork you use to eat dinner. At one end is a handle, and at the other end are two prongs for spearing food. Except on the antibodies these prongs do not spear food. They spear antigens such as pieces of flu virus instead.

It would be great if the antibodies could storm the blood vessel walls and somehow force them to open a hole large enough to free the trapped lymphocyte. But they don't. Just as a carpenter would not use a dinner fork to drill holes in a wall, the immune system does not use antibodies to drill holes in the blood vessels. Antibodies have no direct effect on the vessel walls, but they do recruit cells that can open the wall. Let's see how they do it.

Basophils and Mast Cells

The cells the antibodies recruit are called *mast cells* and *basophils*. For simplicity, we'll refer to them both as mast cells. Like the other cells of the immune army, the mast cells swim lazily in the bloodstream, holding onto their antibody–forks like Goldilocks's three bears clutching their porridge spoons. And just like Goldilocks being awakened by the three furious bears, the mast cells are awakened to frenzied activity when the fork–antibodies they hold spear the flu virus.

Although comparing the mast cells to the three sleeping bears helps us understand how these cells interact with antibodies, we have to adopt another image to understand what the mast cells do next. Once awakened, the mast cells begin to act like immense underwater storage tanks filled with chemicals. And that's exactly what they are.

The excited mast cells release clouds of stored chemicals into the bloodstream, chemicals that dilate the blood vessels, turning the tough little tubes into large, flaccid ones that closely resemble a boiled bratwurst. The dilated vessels develop holes large enough for lymphocytes to escape through, freeing them to pursue and destroy flu viruses outside the blood vessels.

From T Lymphocytes to B lymphocytes to antibodies to mast cells to chemicals, so far our journey through the immune system has been a long one, but at last we have reached our goal of understanding how the hunter–killer lymphocytes are set free. However, to fully understand how the immune system functions, we must go a little further. We must look at one more soldier–cell to see how this vital system gives rise to allergy.

No Brakes

Imagine yourself driving down a steep mountain road. As you follow the tortuous twists and turns of the roadway, you realize your car is traveling dangerously fast. You step on the brakes, but the car continues to gain speed. Frantically, you pump the pedal with your foot, but there's no response—you have no brakes. Moments later, like a runaway train, your car plunges off the mountain road, carrying you to a fiery death.

When fighting infection, your immune system is like this car hurtling down a mountain road. Stimulated into action by an invading virus, hunter–killer T lymphocytes are dividing at breakneck speed, B lymphocytes are spitting out hordes of antibodies, mast cells are dumping hole-opening chemicals all over your blood vessel walls. If there were no way to stop this frantic activity, you would be found in bed the next morning, cold, pale, and dead, with every blood vessel and every pool of body fluid packed with lymphocytes. All the energy you need for living and breathing would have been sucked up to produce this stupendous mass of vessel-clogging immune cells.

Just like your runaway car, this runaway immune system also needs brakes. The brakes for your immune system are supplied by the *suppressor lymphocyte*, the only immune cell with common sense. It works by allowing only a certain number of activated T and B lymphocytes to be produced at one time. By preventing overproduction, the suppressor lymphocyte ensures that only those lymphocytes necessary to defeat the flu virus are produced so that you can survive both the infection and the immune system's response to it.

Into Every Life a Little Rain Must Fall

Ironically, although your life would be impossible without the immune system's germ-killing power, when it fights germs it makes you sick. That's why you feel horrible when you are infected by the flu or a cold virus. To understand how an illness develops, and the immune system's role in making you feel miserable, let's go back to our example of the flu virus infection.

As the mast cell's chemicals dilate the blood vessels and open the holes in their walls, the huge lymphocytes squeeze through in pursuit of the flu virus. However, as the lymphocytes leave the blood vessel, fluid from the bloodstream also gushes through the walls. This happens because the bloodstream is like the plumbing in your house. As pressure in your plumbing system forces the water to run through the water pipes, blood is forced through the blood vessels by the powerful pumping action of the heart.

If you punched a hole in one of the pipes, your plumbing would spring a leak, and the same thing happens when the mast cells punch holes in your blood vessels—blood spurts through the large holes that allow the lymphocytes to escape.

Before the holes open, only a little fluid leaks from the blood vessels. After they open, blood fluid spurts into the areas around the blood vessels, flooding them and making them waterlogged and bloated.

The fluid that escapes and pools around the blood vessels is called edema fluid, and its effects depend on where it accumulates. If it escapes into the lungs, the fluid narrows the air passages, and as the breath travels through the constricted air passages, it produces the wheezing of asthma; this same edema fluid induces chest pain as it squeezes nerve fibers in that area. In the stomach, edema causes burning or cramping, and in the colon, cramps and diarrhea. In the muscles and joints, it causes pain similar to that felt by arthritis sufferers.

In the nose, edema fluid causes congestion, and as it pools and swells the membranes of the sinus cavities, it brings on the pressure-filled pain of sinus headache. In the head, the edema fluid crowds the blood vessels, causing the surges of blood pumping through the blood vessels to set off the throbbing pain of a migraine headache.

And if you think that wheezing, chest pain, joint and muscle aches, diarrhea, abdominal pain, and sinus and migraine headaches are enough misery for the immune system to cause as it sweeps your body clean of the flu virus, you are wrong. You see, the hole-opening chemicals are not the only load carried by the mast cells; they carry much more.

When the mast cells disgorge the hole openers, they also unleash chemicals to make you tired and feverish and chemicals to increase the pain produced by the accumulation of edema. As if the edema needed help!

Now you know why you feel so lousy when you have a virus infection like the flu. It isn't the flu virus that makes your nose run, your throat sore, and your stomach nauseous, it's your body's response to this virus. Why does this vital mast cell cause such misery? I don't know why the great architect of the immune system decided to have the

mast cell produce these devilish chemicals—I wouldn't
have if I been the designer (though I have to admit I was
never asked).

I hope our exploration of the immune system gave you
some insight into how it works. I realize my example is a
simplified picture of how it functions and does not take
into account many important cells and chemicals that contribute to the immune response to germs. But this picture
makes this complicated system more understandable for
me, and I hope it does for you as well. If so, we can take
this knowledge to the next step in our journey as we
explore how the immune system gives rise to allergy in the
following chapter.

How Allergy Causes Headaches

Now that we know a little about how the immune system works to fight off things like flu germs, we can attempt to understand how it brings on allergy-related illnesses like headaches. So turn off the TV, get comfortable in your reading chair, and let's give it a shot.

Why Do We Suffer from Allergic Headaches?

We suffer from allergic headaches because only one cell in the immune system possesses common sense. The rest heedlessly pursue their tasks without giving any thought to the consequences of their actions, and that leads to complications. To understand these complications, we must continue our examination of the immune system and see how this careless pursuit of germs causes allergic headaches.

The Scout

We discussed how the antigen-presenting cell acts as the scout for your underwater immune army. Imagine it swimming along through your bloodstream as you take a refreshing stroll on a sunny day in autumn. All around you, ragweed plants are releasing enormous clouds of pollen into the warm breezes as you enjoy the brisk fall air. As you inhale, you draw its pleasant fragrance into your nose and lungs. Unfortunately, you also inhale the ragweed pollen floating in the air.

The air you take in does not flow gently through your nose like a quiet stream meandering to the sea. No, it rushes in like a turbulent mountain stream, smashing bits of ragweed pollen against your nasal membranes. These membranes are covered with a sticky mucus that traps the ragweed pollen like fly paper traps insects.

This sticky mucus continually cleans the nose of dirt and pollen by flowing out the nostrils, where we remove it by blowing our nose, or by draining down the back of the throat, where we swallow it as postnasal drip. Once swallowed, some of the ragweed survives the acid and enzymes of the intestinal tract and ends up in the body fluid, and from there it enters the bloodstream.

Some of the pollen you inhale from the air escapes harmlessly when you exhale, but some remains in the nose and lungs, dissolved in nasal and bronchial fluid, and from there it gains entrance to the body and joins the ragweed absorbed from the intestine.

After being absorbed through the lungs, nose, and intestines, the ragweed pollen that once floated lazily in the air now drifts innocently in your bloodstream. There it crosses the path of the ever-vigilant antigen-presenting cell, the scout of the immune army.

The cell grabs a piece of the ragweed pollen, examines it suspiciously, and decides that the pollen is a stranger—foreign to the body. For all the antigen-presenting cell knows, it may be part of an invading army of infecting viruses.

Now this cell is no mental giant. If there were a school for cells, it would never get past kindergarten; it probably wouldn't even be able to find its seat in the classroom or learn to raise its hand for permission to go to the lavatory.

Because it lacks good common sense, it reacts as if the harmlessly drifting ragweed were a dangerous infection.

Clutching the piece of ragweed, the antigen-presenting cell races off, frantically searching the bloodstream for a T lymphocyte that can fight the threatening invasion of ragweed pollen (which has no desire to invade anyone, but just landed in the wrong place after its journey through the autumn air).

The Lymphocytes

If there were no T lymphocytes that specialized in the destruction of ragweed invaders, our story would end happily right here—there would be no allergy. Unfortunately, it doesn't happen that way. For some poorly understood reason, all of us, whether allergic or nonallergic, have lymphocytes that specialize in combatting harmless ragweed pollen. In the scheme of life, this is like a regular army having soldiers that specialize in fighting babies in diapers.

The T cells that specialize in fighting ragweed have no more sense than the antigen-presenting cell. When awakened by this cell, they go into frenzied reproduction, churning out son and daughter T lymphocytes dedicated to defeating the hapless bits of ragweed pollen absorbed from the nose, lungs, and intestinal tract. And finding that the ragweed has slipped out of the bloodstream into the body tissues, the hunter–killer T lymphocytes awaken the B lymphocytes, which go into high-speed production of antibodies.

The Mast Cell

Once more, the forklike antibodies tumble through the bloodstream, and once more they are grabbed by the mast cell. When a piece of unsuspecting ragweed pollen wanders by, the antibody tongs spear it, awakening the mast cell to disgorge its load of blood-vessel-dilating and hole-opening chemicals. Once more, as in the fight with the flu virus, fluid gushes out the holes in the vessel walls to swamp the surrounding areas with edema fluid.

What Happens Next?

What happens next depends on where the edema fluid accumulates. Where it accumulates depends on the person affected. We are all unique individuals, and this uniqueness leads to strengths as well as weaknesses. One individual's strength may be a talent for teaching, while another's may be for discovering new materials, or for ministering to the sick. This variety of strengths or talents allows each of us to contribute in a different way to the health of our society.

But we also have weaknesses, and one of them is our susceptibility to illness. We are not all perfectly healthy. Some of us have pancreases that function poorly; we develop diabetes. Some of us have neurotransmitters that function poorly; we develop depression. Some of us have joints that function poorly; we develop arthritis.

These weaknesses may affect the whole body, or they may affect some parts while sparing others. This is particularly true of allergy. Weak blood vessels may allow edema fluid to pool in certain parts of the body, while strong blood vessels prevent the leakage of fluid in other parts. This blend of weak and strong areas determines which illness an allergic person suffers.

Why are some vessels weak? Think of your blood vessels as an oil pipeline stretching over great distances throughout your body. When engineers construct an oil pipeline, no matter how carefully they build, some sections are bound to be defective or to develop defects as they age. Eventually, the defective areas develop leaks and the oil spills, pooling around the pipes like edema fluid pools around your blood vessels.

How does this pattern of weak vessels determine which allergic illness you suffer? If the weak areas in the blood vessels are in the lungs, the edema swelling of the airways causes asthma. If they are in the skin, they cause hives; in the muscles or joints, they cause arthritis-like pain; in the intestines, they cause cramps and diarrhea.

If the weak vessels are in the sinuses, the swelling causes sinus headache. If they are in the blood vessels of the head, the swelling around these blood vessels causes migraine headache. If the swollen areas are around the nerves of the face and scalp, they cause cluster headache.

With this information, we can now define allergy and allergic headaches. *Allergy is a disorder of the immune system that causes swelling of certain areas of the body. Symptoms result based on where the swelling occurs. If it occurs in the sinuses or around the blood vessels or the nerves of the head, it causes sinus, migraine, or cluster headaches.*

Why Are Some People Allergic and Others Not Allergic?

To answer this question we must return to the thesis set forth at the beginning of this chapter: We suffer from allergy because only one cell in the immune system possesses common sense. That cell, of course, is the suppressor lymphocyte, and it is the strength (or weakness) of this cell that determines whether or not a person is allergic.

We watched the antigen-presenting cell float mindlessly through the bloodstream, searching for deadly germs and harmless ragweed with equal dedication. We also watched the T and B lymphocytes hysterically divide, multiply, and spit out chemicals and antibodies to fight both harmful germs and harmless ragweed pollen with the same mindless determination. Finally, we watched the heedless mast cell behave like a ruptured storage tank, dumping vessel-dilating and hole-opening chemicals on vessel walls everywhere in the bloodstream.

All the time this is happening, the suppressor lymphocyte scrutinizes these busy cells, encouraging the T cells to fight the flu germs and discouraging them from fighting ragweed. Cries of "Go get 'em!" and "Now cut that out!"

ring clearly throughout the bloodstream as the constant vigilance of this marvelous cell makes life possible.

Can you guess what would happen if the suppressor lymphocyte failed completely? Without its wise guidance, the immune system would run totally out of control and make a frightful mess. And before long, you would die.

But what if, instead of failing completely, the suppressor lymphocyte becomes only partially disabled? It would still control the immune system, especially the all-important disease-fighting cells. If it didn't, you couldn't exist. But it might become too weak to stop the cells that fight ragweed pollen. If so, the immune system would mount a completely unnecessary but vicious attack against ragweed pollen, causing you to sneeze, wheeze, and suffer headache pain. In other words, you would be allergic.

There is evidence that this happens. In people with allergy, it seems, the harmless ragweed pollen is able to exert a power it does not even want—the power to cause sinus, migraine, and cluster headaches.

How Do You Tell Which Type of Headache You Have?

With what we have learned so far, we have been able to make some educated guesses about the role of allergy in the formation of sinus, migraine, and cluster headaches. But what exactly are these headaches? How do we recognize them? Since each of these headaches has distinct and different symptoms (and we sound smarter if we know how to tell one from another), let's examine them.

The medical textbook descriptions for each of these headache types are long and complicated, but they can also be described simply. As an allergist treating hundreds of new patients each year for these headaches, and noticing how one type of headache often blends into another, making an exact distinction between them of questionable value, I prefer the simple version.

THE MIGRAINE HEADACHE. Almost without exception, those who suffer migraine headache complain of its throbbing pain. The throbbing is caused by a swamp of edema fluid surrounding the dilated blood vessels in the head. As the powerful pumping of the heart repetitively forces blood through these vessels, they throb with pain in tune with the heartbeat.

Where this pain strikes depends on the location of the weak vessels. If they lie on the forehead, the front of the head pulsates with pain. If they lie over one of the temples, the throbbing is felt on the side involved. If all the vessels on one side of the head are affected, that side pounds with pain from front to back; if all the blood vessels of the head are involved, the whole head throbs with pain.

Therefore, the essential characteristic of a migraine headache is throbbing—and often severe—head pain.

CLUSTER HEADACHES. The pain associated with cluster headaches differs from that of migraine in a couple of ways. One way is its severity. Although migraine headache sufferers experience cruel pain, a more fitting adjective to describe the pain of cluster headache is *vicious*.

I suspect this pain is so devastating because it involves the nerves of the face and scalp that carry the sensation of pain to the brain. How efficient these nerves must be when they report to the brain's pain center that they themselves are in pain.

No patient is able to describe this pain accurately. Typically, they report that they feel neither throbbing nor overwhelming pressure (as in sinus headache). This nonspecific description, along with the severity of pain, points to a cluster headache.

There is one other characteristic of cluster headache. Because the nerves of the face and scalp lie just beneath the skin, the cluster headache sufferer feels the pain near the surface of the skin. Whereas patients can only vaguely describe the location of migraine and sinus headaches ("behind my eyes" or "in my forehead"), those with cluster headaches can point to the exact spot where their pain is located. They will often use a finger to draw the path of this pain across their face or scalp.

Where does the name "cluster" come from? In medicine, the name properly applies to headaches that typically affect men with an excruciating pain that strikes frequently and repetitively—a cluster of headaches—and then disappears, only to resurface at another time. They usually strike during the spring and fall pollen seasons, and the pain usually involves one side of the head and is often accompanied by nasal stuffiness and tearing of the eye.

I believe that this headache arises from the nerves supplying the face. I also believe these same nerves are involved in the severe headache my patients describe. Because "nerve headache" is an awkward name, as awkward as calling migraines "blood vessel headaches," I have appropriated the name cluster headache to describe this intensely painful headache.

THE SINUS HEADACHE. Sinus headaches arise in the same way that migraine and cluster headaches do, but the target is not the blood vessels or nerves of the head but the sinus membranes. The blood vessels there dilate and leak edema fluid into the sinus membranes, which swell painfully. This swelling is felt as constant, painful pressure.

WHY DOES A SINUS HEADACHE HURT? Why does swelling and edema of the sinus membrane cause such pain? I suspect it's because the architect of humanity decided to install the sinuses in holes drilled in our skull.

I've often tried to think of a good reason for having our sinuses in holes in our skulls, but I've only been able to come up with fanciful explanations. Perhaps we humans are descended from birds and our sinus cavities are a genetic mutation of their bones, which I understand are full of holes. Makes me think the term "bird brain" is more truth than insult. Whatever the reason, that's where they are.

Because the sinuses are encased in bone, there is no room for them to expand when they swell. It is like trying to blow up a balloon inside a soda bottle. No matter how hard you blow, no matter how much pressure you exert, there is no room for the balloon to expand. In sinus headache, it is the pressure exerted on the sinus walls that causes the pain.

WHERE DO YOU FEEL THE PAIN OF A SINUS HEADACHE? The sinus cavities are located in the bone in your forehead (the frontal sinuses), the bone of your cheeks (the maxillary sinuses), and the bone between your eyes (the ethmoid sinuses). Depending on which sinuses are swollen, you feel the pressure-pain of a sinus headache in your forehead, your cheekbones, or between or behind your eyes.

In these areas, other conditions can cause similar pain. Illnesses of the eye can cause eye pain; tension can often cause forehead pain; and dental problems can cause cheek pain that radiates to the temples if the temporomandibular joint (TMJ) is affected.

Be sure to see your primary doctor so he or she can try to diagnose the true cause. See an eye doctor or dentist, or any other specialist your doctor recommends; use antibiotics if a sinus infection is suspected. If these measures do not relieve your pain, suspect allergic sinus headaches.

Determining whether your pain is due to an allergic swelling of your sinuses is sometimes difficult because other conditions will cause similar pain in the same areas. Diagnosis is even more difficult if the sinus pain decides to spare the forehead, cheeks, and eyes and appear somewhere else.

To understand how this happens, imagine you are calling a friend two blocks away and the telephone is answered, not by your friend, and not even by a person two blocks away, but by a stranger in a town you've never heard of five hundred miles away. "Aha," you say. "Darned wires must be crossed." Your telephone signal must have gone through the wrong line and ended up at a phone far from its intended destination.

The same thing happens with pain impulses. The frontal sinus in your forehead wants to tell you it hurts, so it sends a pain impulse to your brain. When it gets to your brain, if, instead of stimulating the brain cells that signal forehead pain, it takes a wrong turn and shoots to the brain cells that signal pain on the top of the head, you end up with a headache that feels like you're wearing a skullcap two sizes too small. Or it may notify the cells that signal pain in the back of your head, or in the temples, and make you think you have a tension headache. It can even make you feel you have jaw or tooth pain, like a TMJ or dental headache.

Headache sufferers frequently feel pain in areas far from where the pain actually originates. When this happens, the confused patient may travel from primary doctor to neurologist, psychologist, dentist, or orthodontist without anyone realizing the pain is originating from an allergic reaction in the sinus cavities.

The patient is confused, the doctor is confused. If you are the patient and want to end this confusion (who wouldn't?), suspect that allergy may be causing the pain. To do this, you will need to have some clues, and we will discuss some you can use in the next chapter. But first I want to make a couple of other observations related to sinus headache.

A NOTE ABOUT TEETER-TOTTERS. I am confused by something I have noticed on occasions too numerous to count. Two symptoms, nasal stuffiness and sinus headache, often act like two children on a teeter-totter, where one child must be on the ground for the other child to be up in the air. When a patient's nose is completely blocked by allergic swelling (the child up in the air), headaches seldom occur (the child on the ground). Conversely, the more open the nose, the more likely the patient will suffer from head pain.

This teeter-totter effect accounts for the many patients we see in the fall with no nasal stuffiness or sneezing, but with severe sinus, migraine, and cluster headaches. No wonder these miserable people seldom realize ragweed causes their pain.

A REFLECTION ON ABSORPTION. For purposes of our discussion, absorption means to move into the body, from the nose, lungs, or intestinal tract, an inhaled or swallowed particle that was originally in the diet or the environment.

Most people can easily understand that allergy causes a sinus headache. After all, aren't the sinuses in the nose, and don't they receive a large dose of the ragweed pollen that causes the nose to swell? However, the same people have trouble believing that pollen causes the migraine and cluster headaches that occur in blood vessels and nerves far removed from the nose.

It does. Ragweed pollen is absorbed from the nose, lungs, and intestinal tract and circulates through the bloodstream, ultimately reaching the blood vessels and nerves of the head, where it can stimulate the pain of migraine and cluster headache. Therefore, when you think of allergic headaches, don't confine your thinking to sinus headaches. We frequently see patients with combined sinus, migraine, and cluster headache, and we also see patients with the latter two with no associated sinus headache. Ragweed pollen causes all three headaches.

There I go talking about ragweed again. I feel like the kindergarten teacher who continually picks on one child. In our discussion of allergic headaches, we repeatedly blamed fall season ragweed pollen for sinus, migraine, and cluster headaches. Ragweed frequently causes these headaches, but it is not the only culprit. In spring, tree pollen causes headaches, and in midsummer, grass pollen does the same. In late fall, outdoor mold is often to blame, and in winter, house dust mite and indoor mold combine to provoke cluster, migraine, and sinus headaches.

This need not be so. If people recognize that allergy may be the reason they are having headaches, and that allergy treatment will soothe their pain, they can find relief. In the next chapter, we will discuss some clues that will help you determine if allergy is causing your headaches.

Recognizing Allergy as a Cause of Headaches

If I cannot teach you to recognize allergy as a possible cause of your headaches, I cannot help you. Unless you suspect allergy, you cannot benefit from the relief allergy treatment offers and will continue to suffer this painful affliction.

But how do you recognize allergy? Short of divine inspiration striking like a lightning bolt, you must search for clues that point to this diagnosis. Fortunately, there are clues, and the best clue is the other symptoms that accompany headaches. If these symptoms are due to allergy, it is likely that the headaches are also caused by allergy.

To make use of this clue, you must first know about allergic illness. Although this might seem to be a difficult task, it really isn't. When I give a lecture on allergy, I tell my audience a story to help them recognize symptoms that point to this diagnosis. The story may also help you.

A Spaceship Lands

The tale unfolds in a public park, where you are enjoying a picnic with your spouse, your two-month-old baby, three-year-old daughter, and sixteen-year-old son. Just as you finish grilling the hot dogs, twenty feet away lands a flying saucer. A door opens in its silvery side, and out bounces a large, green alien. Raising an armlike appendage in a gesture of friendship, it approaches your family.

The alien mumbles something unintelligible into a machine that translates its rumbling language. Speaking with a midwest accent (my story, I choose the accent), the machine says, "Hello, I come in peace from the star system Alpha Something-or-Other." (I also pick the place.)

"Hello," you answer in your intelligent, cultivated speaking voice. "You are welcome here. Can I help you?"

"Yes, you can," the alien rumbles. "I was sent by my world to count the number of animal species on this planet." It goes on to say that in your family gathering it counts four different species.

Pointing to you and your spouse, it lifts its arm to your height and says, "You two are this tall and speak intelligently. You are one species. The short species you hold in your arms speaks with a squalling noise." Lowering its hand to your three-year-old's height, it continues: "This creature is this tall, and it chatters continually, so it must be another species. And this last creature (pointing to your sixteen-year-old son and raising its hand to his height) is this tall, and its language is a series of grunts."

"Oh, no," you retort, stifling a laugh at the alien's mistake (you have been taught not to laugh at other's mistakes). "I'm afraid you're wrong. We are all of one species, and the differences you see are due to our different ages. My spouse and I are full grown and speak as adults. The child we hold is very young and can only cry at her stage of life. Our three-year-old is just developing language skills and speaks rapidly and incessantly as she practices these skills."

You realize that explaining the sixteen-year-old will be more difficult, but you try. "When the males of our race reach the teenage years, they develop a strange illness. Pronounced weakness causes their heads to slump forward on their shoulders and forces them to lean against any available surface. They also temporarily lose their language skills and are able to communicate with adults only in grunts."

The Point of the Story

Things that seem exceedingly complicated are often very simple. The alien thought your family gathering represented a complicated mixture of different species; you knew it represented only one species. The alien was confused by the different sizes and speech patterns of your family members; you knew these differences were due to the difference in ages. The reason for the size and language differences was not complicated. It was simple.

Allergy is also simple, although it may appear complicated. Once we understand the immune system and how it spawns allergy, the basic simplicity of this seemingly complicated illness emerges from the mystery and confusion surrounding it. If we hold the key to this simplicity, recognizing allergy becomes much easier.

(Remember, if you realize that some of your symptoms are caused by allergy, you have a valuable clue that your headaches are also caused by allergy.)

Simplifying Allergy

In the previous chapter, we discussed how allergic illness can be regarded as edema swelling brought on by the immune system. We also learned that the type of allergic illness that results depends upon where the edema swelling is located: if it occurs in the lungs, it causes asthma; in the skin, it causes hives; in the muscles or joints, it causes arthritis-like pain; in the stomach or intestines, it causes cramps and diarrhea. And finally, we learned that it causes a different type of headache depending upon which area of the head is involved: the sinuses (sinus headache), the blood vessels (migraine headache), or the nerves of the face and scalp (cluster headache).

I am sure there are more complicated definitions of allergy, but they provide no better understanding. Let others make their definitions complicated; you and I will keep ours simple and understandable.

Taking the Complexity Out of Allergy Diagnosis

An example of how a simple definition of allergy makes diagnosing allergy easier occurred recently. Liz, who is one of the excellent young doctors in family practice training programs in our area, was spending two weeks in our office learning about allergy. She and I had examined Rosie, a forty-five-year-old patient sent to me by her internist for diagnosis of her chronic cough.

Rosie also suffered periods when hives erupted on her skin. In addition, she told us about the extensive tests she had undergone two years earlier and her multiple consultations with various doctors when, for a period of months, she completely lost her voice.

When we asked about headaches, she said they bothered her rarely, but that when they occurred, the pain was overwhelming. Twice a year, a week-long bout of this pain literally knocked her flat in bed. Extensive tests and neurological consultations had been unable to determine a cause for these excruciating headaches.

Then, almost as an afterthought, she related that she often ran out of breath when she climbed stairs. She said it felt as if something were blocking her air passages.

After interviewing Rosie, Liz and I were discussing her case, and I asked Liz if she found Rosie's story confusing.

"Yes, I do," she answered. "All these various symptoms happening to the same patient? Hives, voice loss, stuffy nose, severe headaches, breathing difficulty with exercise." With a puzzled look, she suggested a possible reason,

"Perhaps these many unrelated symptoms exist only in her mind, brought on by psychological stress and anxiety."

"That may be so, Liz," I said. "But before we blame stress and anxiety, let's see if allergy might be an alternative explanation."

Liz and I had already discussed allergy's nasty habit of causing swelling in various areas of the body. To my mind, Rosie's story dramatized this well.

"Liz, what if all of Rosie's symptoms were caused by the same disease? Her current problem of persistent coughing could be caused by an immune reaction to allergy, and you can think of it as having a hive in her upper airway that causes a ticklish sensation, which she relieves by coughing. You noticed that she pointed to an area at the base of her neck when she described the tickle-cough."

I saw that Liz was grasping the point I was making. I went on to say, "If the hive had been higher in the respiratory tract, in the throat, it could swell her vocal cords and she would lose her voice in exactly the manner she described. Swelling lower in the respiratory tract, in the chest, would block some of the air passages of her lungs, and she would experience shortness of breath as she climbed stairs or did other exercises."

Liz agreed with this possibility. "Then all her various symptoms are due to the same cause, an allergic swelling in different areas of her respiratory tract," she said. "That means her symptoms are predictable and not strange. They logically center in the areas where the swellings occur."

"That's my interpretation of her symptoms," I replied, pleased at Liz's realization that Rosie's many different symptoms came from the same source. "Her hives are also caused by this same allergic swelling appearing on her skin and are a good sign that swelling is occurring in her respiratory tract."

"What about the headaches she experiences?" Liz asked.

"If you visualized these hives as swellings in her sinus cavities, the resulting pressure would cause a severe headache," I replied.

Some Lessons from Rosie's Story

Besides the obvious lesson that diagnosing allergy is not difficult, if you think of it as causing swelling in different areas of the body, Rosie's story teaches a number of other lessons.

- Allergy can *begin* at any time of life—Rosie's cough started recently, but her headaches and hives have bothered her for years. Thus, all symptoms need not develop at the same time.

- As in Rosie's story, allergy often *skips* from one part of the body to another, swelling shut the eustachian tube and causing ear infections in the seven-year-old, swelling the skin and causing hives in the seventeen-year-old, and swelling the blood vessels of the head and causing migraine headaches in the seventy-year-old.

- The swelling of *hives* on the skin is an excellent indication that there is swelling inside the body, but don't be fooled if a person with headaches has no skin swelling. Many patients with allergic migraine and sinus headache do not have hives, although they may develop them years after the headaches start.

- Allergy symptoms may *disappear* for years and *reappear* in their old form or as new symptoms, as Rosie's did. The infant's colic may return as the teenager's hives or as the adult's headache.

- Whether allergic symptoms are single or multiple, most are caused by *swelling* in the affected areas.

Allergy is a malicious little gremlin that likes to hide its deviousness behind a smokescreen of seeming complexity. It causes symptoms that can start at any time of life, skip from place to place in the body, and disappear and reappear over the years. It does this to confuse you and prevent you from realizing that, far from being complex, its effects can be easy to recognize. All you need is some knowledge of allergy and immunology.

Some Allergic Headaches Are Easy To Recognize

The diagnosis of allergic headaches is greatly simplified when they are accompanied by other symptoms that are plainly and unarguably caused by allergy. When warm summer breezes carry their loads of pollen to the unfortunate person afflicted with hay fever, miserable symptoms erupt. They include itching skin, dripping nose, swollen eyes, and of course, the always distressing sneezing. That the peak number of headaches occurring during the summer are due to pollen few would doubt.

Also easy to recognize is the headache that appears during an attack of hives in a person allergic to peanuts who has eaten peanut butter, or the headache that appears along with an episode of cramping and diarrhea in a person allergic to shrimp who has unwisely eaten a shrimp cocktail. Also, there is little reason to doubt the presence of allergy when people allergic to cats and dogs react with headaches while visiting a home where these animals are kept as pets.

Patients who react to pollen, peanut, shrimp, dog, and cat exposures are unlucky to be plagued with these allergies but fortunate that the causes of their headaches are so obvious. Because the causes are not in doubt, sufferers can identify the origins of their discomfort, and because the causes are known, they can be treated.

Some Allergic Headaches Are Harder To Recognize

Sometimes the person suffering from headaches never even considers allergy as a cause. This happens frequently when the headaches are accompanied by symptoms that are not generally known to be caused by allergy. In these cases, the affected person will not find the cause in the shrimp cocktail or the jar of peanut butter. Nor do the headaches closely relate to the summer pollen season or to exposure to the cat or dog. The unfortunate sufferer is baffled by these mysterious head pains and will not seek the effective help that allergy treatment provides.

When allergy's role in headaches is hidden, its presence can often be uncovered by searching for clues. The best clue is the presence of other allergic illnesses, even those usually not thought to be caused by allergy. This clue can be found in: *(1)* symptoms affecting the person today (history of present illness); *(2)* symptoms that affected the person in the past (past history); *(3)* symptoms affecting biologically related relatives (family history).

Symptoms Affecting the Person Today

Often, headaches are accompanied by symptoms that, for the knowledgeable person, strongly point to allergy. As discussed earlier, they may be accompanied by hives on the skin and various symptoms that can be explained as hivelike swellings in the air passages, muscles, or intestines. To be more specific, head pain may be accompanied by asthma, arthralgia, or abdominal cramps and diarrhea.

When headaches are accompanied by symptoms that are best explained as swellings on the skin or in the body, it is easy to suspect there is similar swelling in the sinuses or in the nerves and blood vessels of the head. In these cases, the associated symptoms will point to allergy as a cause of the headaches like a traffic cop points the way at a busy intersection.

In harder-to-recognize allergic illnesses, symptoms often act like virus infections. Because the attention of the doctor or patient is wholly focused on treating viral illnesses, they miss the allergy that is aggravating the illness. This often happens because the untreated allergic person is unusually susceptible to virus infections. To make things worse, each of these recurrent virus infections causes allergy to flare up.

For example, we have all experienced viral infections like the common cold or the flu. With these regrettable conditions, our noses drip, our throats and ears ache, our eyes burn, and we cough and sneeze and wheeze. Perhaps our stomachs churn and our trips to the toilet are frequent. Doctors call these illnesses by such names as upper respiratory infections or abdominal viral illnesses, and the lay public calls them colds or the stomach flu. When they occur infrequently—once or twice a year—there is no reason to suspect allergy. However, when they keep returning and the symptoms are persistent, it is likely due to this peculiar combination of viruses and allergy.

Why should a person have ten colds a winter, a sore throat every two weeks, abdominal cramps and diarrhea month after month? These are all symptoms that virus colds and flu cause, but because they persist an unreasonable length of time and return far too often, more than a simple, uncomplicated virus is involved. If a good examination by the primary doctor shows no other underlying cause, suspect the allergy–virus combination.

That allergy and viral illnesses act the same is not surprising. As we discussed, when a virus invades the body, its invasion triggers a vicious attack by the immune system like the bell in a heavyweight boxing match triggers the boxers to attack each other. And just as the winner of a heavyweight fight is bruised and battered during the match, so is the winner of the immune-versus-virus match.

The immune system shares in this battering, and the immune cell that often pays the highest price for the victory is the suppressor lymphocyte. Weakened by the fight with the virus, it loses its ability to control the immune system and suppress it when it attacks harmless allergens. Without the calming influence of the weakened suppressor lymphocyte, the immune T and B lymphocytes and the mast cells attack pollens, dust mites, molds, animal danders, and foods. The affected person suffers the painful and uncomfortable effects of the vasodilation and edema resulting from this allergic response.

It often takes weeks for the suppressor lymphocyte to recover and stop the runaway lymphocytes and mast cells so the symptoms of cough, runny nose, wheezing, headaches, and other unpleasant miseries of allergy can subside. Often, before the suppressor lymphocyte recovers, it is hit by another virus, usually one so weak itself that it would not even bother the nonallergic person.

Sometimes the suppressor lymphocyte does not recover, and the temporary state of allergy that follows a virus infection becomes permanent. Symptoms like wheezing, nasal stuffiness, and headaches last for years. That's why allergic patients so often date the onset of their allergic illness to a time when they suffered a bad cold.

Which allergic illnesses act like viral illnesses? The following is a partial list:

- *Head*—Recurrent sore throats and throat tightness; itching and/or burning eyes; recurrent earaches and ear infections; recurrent and persistent colds.

- *Chest*—Recurrent chest pains; recurrent chest colds, shortness of breath, and wheezing.

- *Abdomen*—Recurrent abdominal pain and/or cramping; recurrent loose stools and/or diarrhea (often called spastic colon).

Therefore, in looking for signs that allergy may be causing headaches, don't overlook illnesses that appear to be caused by viruses if the illnesses are persistent and recurrent. They are an excellent sign that allergy is present and may be causing headaches.

Searching for Allergy in Past Illnesses

Many times patients suffering from headaches have no other symptoms. Are their headaches caused by allergy?

One way to decide whether allergy could be the cause is to search the patient's memory for past illnesses caused by allergy. Remember, the gremlin of allergy may have struck in the past, leaving a clue to his involvement in today's headaches like a criminal's past record alerts a detective to his recent crimes.

This is practical advice. Many of my patients with headaches are currently free of allergic symptoms but suffered allergic illnesses earlier in life. Because they have not had symptoms for many years, they make the mistake of believing they are free of allergy—thinking it has "gone away."

This frequently turns out not to be the case. Like a chameleon changes its color, their allergy has changed its symptoms. It has returned in the form of headaches.

Laura's Story

An example of this chameleon-like phenomenon (and an example of the value of searching a patient's past history) is the story of Laura. As a baby, she cried and squirmed with colic until she was four months old. She had frequent and recurrent ear infections starting at three months of age and continuing until she was seven years old. Her asthma started when she was four and continued until age twelve. Then, for thirteen years, she was free of any allergy symptoms.

When she initially visited me for consultation, she was twenty-five years old, had recently had a baby, and was an accountant for a CPA firm. Her headaches had started nine months prior to her first visit, after years free of illness.

"Well, Laura, what brings you to see me?" I asked.

"My doctor insisted I see you because of my headaches," she answered, with a note of doubt in her voice that was explained by what she said next: "I don't think my headaches are allergic. I used to have allergies when I was a child, but they are all gone now."

Laura's response is typical of many patients. She suffered from allergy in the past but believed allergy had "gone away." But it didn't go away. It just changed, much like the weather changes from sunny to rainy, from balmy to cold.

As a child, Laura's obvious allergy caused her colic, asthma, and ear infections. As an adult, it is no longer obvious, but it still causes pain and discomfort—her headaches. If Laura had realized the headaches were caused by allergy, she could have received effective treatment months earlier.

The moral of Laura's story is, if you want to find clues to the cause of this year's headaches, look for allergic illnesses that occurred in past years.

What If There Is No Past History of Allergy?

People with allergic headaches may never have experienced allergic illness of any type before their headaches began. Allergy symptoms can start at any time of life, and headaches may be the first symptom to appear. Hence, many headache sufferers do not have previous symptoms as a clue to use in searching for the cause of their irritating pain.

However, all is not lost. Allergy tends to run in families, and looking for allergic illnesses in other family members may provide clues to the cause of a person's headaches. A close relative having allergy should suggest this diagnosis in a person suffering allergic headaches. The following story demonstrates this point.

Ben's Story

Ben, a twenty-year-old college student, and his mother were practically dragged into my office. The dragger was his girl friend, whose headaches were being controlled by allergy treatment. She suspected Ben's headaches were also due to allergy.

Ben freely admitted he resented being in my office. "I don't know why I'm here because I don't think my headaches are due to allergy," he stated categorically. I wasn't surprised by Ben's resentment; young men often avoid going to a doctor because they see it as a sign of weakness.

However, Ben reluctantly described his headaches for me, which were occurring daily and were both the throbbing and pressure types—migraine and sinus. They started in the back of his head, traveled over the top of his skull, and burrowed into his forehead and eyes. They were aggravating and often strikingly painful.

Ben's pain was typical of the head pain my patients frequently describe, so I asked his mother if he had ever experienced any other allergic illnesses. She told me he had not. Since he had no other signs of allergy, I asked her about other members of the family.

"My husband has a constant stuffy nose, and we often wonder if allergy might be causing it," she said. "And two of his brothers have bad hay fever. They were both on allergy shots as children and are thinking of starting them again."

The news that Ben was part of a family with allergies considerably increased the likelihood that his headaches were due to allergy. Both Ben and his mother agreed that this was possible, and Ben decided to pursue allergy treatment. On a following visit, I learned our treatment was working well. Ben's headaches were less frequent, and he was pleased with the results. His headaches *were* due to allergy.

Can Headaches Be Due to Allergy If There Is No Present, Past, or Family History of Allergy?

Yes, they can. Although a person may be born with the genetic potential to suffer allergic illnesses, this potential may never be activated, or may be activated much later in life. If the only illness activated is headaches, and the allergic family members never show any symptoms, then there may be no present, past, or family history of allergy.

In these cases, the diagnosis is often overlooked—it's easy to do and no one's fault. But it is unfortunate, because the patient may never receive the relief provided by allergy treatment.

* * *

You cannot be treated for allergy if you are unaware it causes your headaches. Don't overlook its clues. Look at the illnesses that accompany your headaches; they might lead you to consider allergy as the cause. Look at the illnesses you suffered in the past; they may also help. Look at your family history of illnesses; the answer may be there. If these clues don't exist, or if you don't pay attention to the clues that do exist, you or your loved one may be condemned to suffer head pain needlessly.

Both What You Eat and What You Breathe

Thomas Cleary relates an interesting story in his translation of Sun Tzu's ancient classic, *The Art of War*. A lord of China asked a question of a famous doctor who belonged to a family of doctors: Which of the brothers was most skilled in the healing arts and most famed in the community?

This physician, renowned in China for his medical prowess, answered thus (my interpretation of the story):

"My oldest brother recognizes the causes of illness and removes them before they bring illness, so his fame does not travel beyond his own house."

"My second brother cures sickness quickly when it starts, so his fame does not travel beyond the neighborhood."

"As for me, I can neither prevent illness nor cure it when it first arises. However, because I puncture veins, prescribe potions, and massage skin, my name is spoken among the lords from time to time. Therefore, although my skill is the least, my fame is the greatest."[1]

---

[1] From *The Art of War*, by Sun Tzu, translated by Thomas Cleary. © 1988 by Thomas Cleary. Reprinted by arrangement with Shambhala Publications, Inc., 300 Massachusetts Avenue, Boston, Massachusetts 02115.

For any deviation in paraphrasing this story, I extend my apologies to Mr. Cleary and the ancient Chinese philosopher who first narrated this thought-provoking parable. My only excuse is that I am greatly impressed with its enduring wisdom—it is as pertinent today as it was long ago. A doctor with superlative skill in the healing arts should *prevent* illness, not treat its sad consequences.

As Sun Tzu's *The Art of War* stresses the preservation of peace as the cure for war, medicine must stress the preservation of health as the cure for illness. Our fame as doctors is dramatically enhanced as we do battle against the ravages of illness. However, how much less would be our fame but greater our skill if we could prevent it before it affected our patients.

Practitioners in every field of medicine agree with this thinking and strive toward this goal. Those of us who treat allergy are fortunate to have the means to reach it. We know the things that make our patients suffer and can teach our patients to avoid them. We can end their miserable symptoms. We can prevent headaches.

However (you knew there had to be a *however*, didn't you?), this can only happen if people understand the sources of their allergy, the environmental and dietary roots that feed their pain. Further, they must have the desire to change their environment and diet and the ability to do so. Only then can these roots be destroyed.

This is possible. The offenders in the environment and the diet can be identified. Ways to minimize or eliminate their effects are available. However (there's that word again), headache sufferers themselves must change their diet and environment—other than through persuasion and encouragement, no one else can do this job. Fortunately (a much better word), my experience with many patients has repeatedly demonstrated that when they realize the causes of their discomfort, they find ways to fight them. Human resourcefulness and determination are awesome.

Allergic Headaches Come from the Environment

Headaches bring pain and misery. They are devoid of mercy; they are without honor. Even though a man might be strong and courageous, against headaches he is defenseless. And they take equal delight in punishing the weak and frail. They bring days of irritability and crying to the very young, nights of pain and troubled sleep to the elderly. They thrust a harsh tone into a mother's voice and a mean note into a child's response. They diminish the clarity of thought, the caliber of work, and the worth of study.

Where do we look for the roots that nourish these despicable pains? Do we look in old and musty basements, where cobwebs drape from the ceilings and splotches of green and black mold decorate the walls? Yes, the roots are there.

Do we look in swamps and marshes, where green algae floats in the water and decaying vegetation releases its stink to the passing winds. Yes, the roots are there also.

But, the headache sufferer makes a terrible mistake searching for the causes of headaches only in these places of obvious mustiness and decay.

Headache's causes also ride on the warm, scented breezes that delight the senses on a sunny afternoon in May. They float in the still clear air of the Nebraska plains, travel with the cool winds of the Minnesota forests, and live in the air that surrounds your home and yard. They share the air you breathe as you prepare a meal, watch TV, and snore softly at night.

You need not go to some moist, moldy, and creepy place to find the reasons for headaches. The causes are all around—they hide in plain sight. Because you live so intimately with them, you fail to recognize their presence. This can change. If you open your eyes to your environment, find the things that breed headaches and eliminate them, you can make your headaches stop.

Allergic Headaches Come from the Diet

To stop headaches, we must search for the causes not only in the air we breathe, but also in the foods and beverages that nourish us. It is right to expect that our environment causes headaches, but it is wrong to focus on that alone. The diet must also be examined. As living human organisms, we need both food and air; life is impossible without either of them. The need to eat and drink is a vulnerability that headaches exploit to disturb our lives.

Patients with headaches often make the mistake of looking for the cause of head pain only in the diet or only in the environment. This often happens because a book or TV show highlights the pain-causing potential of a particular food or environmental exposure. Focusing so much attention on it makes it seem to be the only important cause. Usually, the food or the exposure is important; the only error in the presentation is the failure to recognize that its subject is but one of the many factors that generate headaches.

Let's not make this mistake. Let's not fixate on only one cause of headaches. Let's scrutinize both the environment and the diet.

How should we look for headache causes in the diet? We should use the same approach we discussed when searching the environment—concentrate on the dramatic as well as the commonplace. We should apply this same principle in scrutinizing our diet.

We tend to search for headache causes in moldy food or foods high in yeast; we look to "fast food" and "junk food"; we look to whatever food or beverage it is currently fashionable to fear or blame. However, when we stop eating these foods and our headaches do not stop, we become confused. This confusion is to be expected.

It arises because some fast foods and junk foods cause headaches, but not all of them do. Moldy and yeasty foods also cause headaches, but little of what we eat is moldy or yeasty. Confusion also arises because many of the foods and beverages that cause headaches are foods that, from early life, we have been taught to regard as essential parts of a balanced diet. How can these foods cause our headaches? Their reputation as healthful and essential allows them to hide the fact that they bring pain under a cloak of respectability.

We are also confused because we expect that unusual or exotic foods cause our headaches. These foods *can* bring pain, so pay attention to their effects when you eat them. However, the foods we eat every day also cause headaches—far more frequently than the rarely eaten foods—so do not ignore their contribution to your pain.

Finally, we are confused if we do not realize how many foods and beverages cause headaches. Because there are so many, it serves little purpose to remove one or two from our diet; those that remain will continue to cause pain. Attacking the problem of food allergy in this hit-or-miss fashion is likely to have little or no effect.

Before you can eliminate the offending foods and beverages from your diet and reduce the dust, molds, pollens, and other elements in the environment, you must know their identity, why they bother you, and how to fight them. In the following chapters, we will explore these issues so that you will have the information you need to attack the problem.

As we explore, open your mind to the idea that your diet and your home are major causes of your headaches. Resist the all too human tendency to defend them; they do you no favors. Only when you recognize their potential for harm will you accept the timeless advice of the ancient Chinese parable and adopt the wisdom of the oldest brother—you will prevent your headaches by removing the things that cause them. The treatment of the physician will no longer be necessary.

Part II
Moisture, Mites, and Mold

Moisture

We humans are an opinionated lot, confident that our assertions are not only correct but also brilliant (as they often aren't). If asked for our opinion on any subject, we reply without hesitation and with absolute certainty. This is especially true when we are asked to expound on the most important aspect of any topic. For instance, if asked what they view as the most important part of an airplane, one person might answer, "The wings, of course. They keep the plane aloft." And another might say, "Without a doubt, the engines. A plane cannot fly without engines."

If asked my opinion, I would say it is neither wings nor engines that are the most essential part. My limited experiences as a passenger have convinced me there is something else even more important.

I am scared stiff of flying—probably because I find it hard to believe that huge metal monster can hurtle down the runway, soar into a steep climb, and not belly flop back to the ground. This suspicion is confirmed each time I travel on a plane by the two loud thumps I hear just after takeoff. The first thump is the sound of the plane hitting the telephone pole at the end of the runway; the second is the sound of one of the engines falling off.

When I inform the flight attendant of these catastrophes, she patiently reassures me that the two thumps I heard were only the sound of the landing gear retracting. But I'm not easily fooled. I wasn't born yesterday.

Which brings me to what I think is the most important part of an airplane. In my opinion, it is the flight attendant who, at the end of the flight, with the utmost kindness and patience, helps pry my clawed fingers away from the armrest.

As these examples illustrate, opinions on what constitutes the most important aspect of any topic, whether airplanes or headaches, can differ markedly from one person to another. That is why I approach with caution the question of utmost significance for those who suffer head pain: Of all the things that contribute to causing headaches, which is the most important?

Since I am just as opinionated as the next person, and equally sure of the correctness of my opinion, which was formed after years of treating patients with headaches, I believe there is only one answer: The most important cause of headaches is moisture.

Why is moisture so important? Because it leads to the humidity that allows house dust mites, mold, yeast, and algae to grow. Although we tend to believe these organisms grow only in the high humidity typical of swampy areas and moldy old houses, they do not require such conditions to proliferate. A more moderate and comfortable forty to fifty percent relative humidity is perfectly adequate. This is the level of humidity found in our homes in summer, and many homes retain this humidity throughout the winter.

Why Is Humidity Troublesome?

There are several reasons why I believe humidity—and the dust mites, mold, algae, and yeast it nurtures—is the prime culprit in causing allergic headaches. First, among our patients, those who live in moist homes seem to suffer more frequent and painful headaches than those who live in drier homes. These headaches are also harder to treat.

When patients complain of daily headaches, I usually find they live in homes with more moisture than patients who suffer weekly or monthly headaches. This same difference exists for patients whose headaches are severely painful when compared with those whose headaches are less severe. Patients with the highest frequency and severity of headaches come from moist homes.

My nurses and I are also convinced that patients who live in very moist environments need more exacting dietary changes and more frequent allergy injections than patients who live in drier surroundings. Thus, even treatment requirements seem to be affected by moisture.

There is a final reason we believe that moisture and the organisms that thrive because of it are predominant causes of headache. When our patients correct these moisture problems, their headaches usually subside.

Beth's Story

Beth's story is a good example of the harmful effects of moisture. I first saw her when she was twenty-six years old, four years after she married and moved to her present home and two years after headaches began to alter her life. Her pain was terrible. No day passed without agonizing pressure in her forehead and behind her eyes, and the feeling that her head would explode. No week passed without her temples throbbing with the pain of migraine headache. She needed relief.

Doctors had tried to help. Beth had consulted two neurologists, who ordered numerous tests in an attempt to find the cause of these frustrating pains. Blood tests were normal. X-rays and brain scans were normal. Medication gave her some relief, as did relaxation therapy and biofeedback, but her painful headaches continued. At the suggestion of her current neurologist, she came to my office to see if I could do anything for her.

When I first saw Beth, I realized she would be difficult to treat but I didn't appreciate how difficult until later.

My staff and I treat many patients with headaches as severe as Beth's, patients who do well with allergy treatment. These patients usually live in damp surroundings, such as a basement apartment or an older home where mold is present. Treatment almost always reduces the frequency and severity of their headaches—but only after the moisture problem is eliminated or reduced.

It was logical to suspect that Beth's daily sinus and weekly migraine headaches were brought on by the moist conditions in her home, moisture that promoted heavy growth of mold, yeast, algae, and house dust mite.

When I questioned Beth, she identified several conditions in her home that signalled mustiness. At our suggestion, she took steps to correct these conditions. She removed the old carpet from her basement and threw away the books that had accumulated there. She gave away most of her plants and stopped using the humidifier.

Unfortunately, despite making these changes, she still suffered daily headaches. Although allergy injections and diet changes helped, they did not completely put an end to her misery.

I was frustrated at being unable to conquer Beth's remaining headaches, and she was depressed because she continued to suffer. We almost stopped the allergy injections and dietary changes a number of times, but decided to persist because they provided some relief, albeit incomplete. Beth and I hoped that continued treatment would increase this relief, as it often does.

Then, after two years of treatment, I saw Beth for an office visit. It was a visit I will never forget. We were reviewing her symptoms over the previous six months, and

I asked, "How are your headaches, Beth?" I wasn't expecting much of a change, so what she said next came as quite a surprise.

"I'm much better, Dr. Walsh," she replied, smiling for the first time that I could remember. "My head hurts only once a week, or so, and the pain is much less severe. It doesn't even wake me up at night."

I was thrilled but puzzled. What had happened? Why this welcome change? When I asked her, she replied, "You kept questioning me about moldiness at home, and my husband and I kept looking for it. Well, we finally found it. It was inside a wall in our bedroom. We smelled something musty on one side of our bedroom, and then I noticed a spot of mold on the wall inside a closet."

Beth told me that her husband had torn out the inside of the wall and found the insulation green with mold. Sometime in the past the roof must have leaked, and water found its way into the wall, causing mold to grow. After the insulation was replaced, Beth began to enjoy days without torment and nights of unbroken sleep. She was tickled to be free of this awful pain, and I was relieved that the cause of her headaches was no longer a mystery.

You might think Beth's story is somewhat unusual because the offending mustiness was hidden inside a wall of her home. However, she is not alone in living with hidden moisture. We frequently see patients whose symptoms turn out to be from similar concealed mustiness. They make me wonder how many other headache sufferers live unsuspectingly with this bothersome problem.

An Unfinished Story

Jack is a new patient to our practice whose headaches are as frequent and painful as Beth's used to be. Like Beth's, his pain occurs daily, but unlike Beth's, it is centered behind his eyes and covers the top of his head like a skullcap designed by the Marquis de Sade. Jack lives in an older mobile home, and I suspect the walls have the same moldy condition that Beth found. I also suspect that musty air from under the mobile home is seeping into it, fostering the growth of dust mites, mold, yeast, and algae, and making him miserable.

Jack and I talked about his home and my concern about its condition. He shares this worry. He plans to move in the near future, and when he does, I expect his headaches will abate as Beth's did.

It was reassuring to know that Jack shared my concern. I have tremendous respect for my patients' opinions because they are so often right. Frequently, I find that they were worried about moisture problems in their homes long before I first mentioned them. They share my suspicions. When their exposure to the mustiness is reduced or eliminated, they almost always find their headaches tapering off. They live with much less pain.

My Story

I have had my own experience with mold in the home. Awhile back, I began to notice a peculiar smell in one of the rooms in our house—the same mustiness you smell on a rainy day in the woods. Now the earthy smell of wet vegetation can be quite pleasant in its proper place—namely, the woods on a rainy day—but not in a bedroom, especially since just being in the room made my nose stuffy. I knew I needed to find the reason for the odor.

Taking no pleasure in the chaos it would create, I decided I would have to tear the Sheetrock off the wall. As soon as I could see inside the wall, the reason for the smell became apparent—moldy, green insulation.

What had caused this to happen? I found the answer in the attic. The strong easterly winds of a winter storm had blown snow through an attic vent and deposited a small white snowdrift over the area where I discovered the moldy insulation. When the sun warmed the attic, the

snow melted and ran down inside the wall, soaking into
the insulation and creating a perfect environment for the
growth of mold—a dark, damp place with no ventilation.

My next problem was to find a way to keep snow from
getting into the attic. I thought I had solved it by placing a
furnace filter over the vent—until I noticed a large wet spot
on the ceiling below the area after a rainstorm. The furnace
filter worked fine for snow, but it did a poor job of keeping
rain from getting into the attic.

As I repainted the ceiling, I rethought my less-than-bril-
liant solution to the problem. The vent is now blocked with
a permanent plywood plug, and a new ridge vent has been
installed to ventilate the attic. And I am praying that this
remedy works.

Another Moisture Source

The moldy wall was not the only part of my home that
had moisture problems. For years, my garage smelled like a
musty graveyard during the spring and fall rainy seasons. I
couldn't understand why. The gutters and downspout did
a good job of channeling the water from the roof into the
back yard and preventing water from penetrating the
garage. Or so I thought.

I found out I was wrong when I decided to investigate
during a heavy downpour. As I walked the yard in my
raincoat and umbrella, I saw that the gutters and downspouts were indeed collecting the rain that fell on the roof
and diverting it to the back yard. However, the landscape
drainage behind the garage was terrible. The water pooled
in the yard, saturating the soil and eventually seeping
under the garage, keeping the floor constantly wet. That's
why the garage smelled so badly.

When I changed the direction of the downspout, allowing the rainwater to flow down a nearby hill, the garage
dried out and stayed dry, even when it rained. There was
another bonus. My basement also smelled better because

the water that collected under the garage had also been seeping into the basement wall, raising the humidity down there to an uncomfortable level.

As my nose unclogged, and I began to enjoy the clean, dry smell of the garage and basement—all due to my excellent detective work, I became quite smug about my keen powers of deduction. It had taken only fifteen years to figure it out.

Look Everywhere for Moisture

So far, the examples I have used are ones where the source of moisture was hidden, but don't be misled by this. Many sources are plainly visible in our everyday surroundings, and I will describe them later. However, the previous examples are relevant because they illustrate the harm caused by exposure to excessive moisture and to the mold (plus algae and yeast) it breeds. A musty environment, whether at home, school, or work, makes headache treatment frustratingly difficult.

If my patients live where there is excessive moisture, I am frequently unable to adequately control the headaches that plague them, despite the powerful weapons given me by medical science. Fortunately, this does not happen often. Most of the patients I treat gain satisfying relief from the dietary changes and allergy injections that are part of the allergist's arsenal. When these measures have poor results, a musty home is usually the problem.

Beth's story illustrates this point. As long as the mustiness was present in her home, her headaches responded poorly to treatment. She continued to suffer despite taking great care to avoid foods that provoke headaches. She continued to suffer despite taking allergy injections to dust mite, mold, and pollen. She continued to suffer despite using many excellent medications. All these potent therapies were no match for the moldy insulation inside her wall.

My practice is filled with countless other examples of headaches due to moisture and the organisms that grow in this dampness. I am reminded of Sue, whose frequent severe headaches also responded to treatment very grudgingly. She was a very caring young mother of two charming little girls, and due to limited skills and the need to be home with her children, she was unemployed and could only afford a basement apartment in an older building.

The rent was cheap; the air was musty. Both Sue and I suspected the apartment was the source of her headaches, but she wasn't able to move until two years after we began allergy treatment, when she remarried and moved to a drier home. While she was living in her apartment, not a day went by without Sue having headaches; on some days the pain was so severe she couldn't function normally and had to lie down. A year after the move, her headaches subsided, occurring only once a week or so, and the pain no longer forced her into bed. They even responded to aspirin. Again, as in Beth's case, Sue's treatment was stymied by excess moisture.

Moisture Headaches Need Not Be Overwhelming

Because I have concentrated on cases where exposure to very high levels of mold and moisture led to frequent and brutal headaches, you may think moisture is not important for patients whose headaches are not as frequent or as severe. This is not so. Eliminating or reducing moisture is equally as effective for those with weekly sinus or monthly migraine headaches as for those whose headaches occur more often. In fact, the results in this less affected group are often surprisingly gratifying.

As a general rule, the less frequent and severe the headaches, the less exposure the patient has to moisture and the easier it is to eliminate. The person with weekly headaches is less likely to live in a basement apartment or a musty mobile home than the person with daily headaches.

He or she is also more likely to gain relief without being forced to move to another home. In many cases, avoiding the basement family room and turning off the humidifier is all that is necessary for medications, diet changes, and allergy injections to be fully effective.

* * *

Whether headaches occur daily or weekly, whether the pain is mild or excruciating, allergy treatment usually provides welcome relief. It works because it attacks the harm caused by the organisms that grow in moisture. The results are even better if dampness is eliminated.

I hope the examples in this chapter will help you understand why I consider moisture the most important factor my patients with headaches must confront. Of course, it is not the only reason for their headaches—animals, pollen, and many foods also provoke headaches, but these exposures are far more obvious than the mustiness that so often hides its presence and is difficult to detect.

One reason problems due to moisture remain so well hidden is that no homeowner wants to believe his or her home could have such problems. When we question them, our patients frequently insist, "My home is dry," or "My basement isn't wet." But you would be wise not to think that way. Recognize that your headaches have a cause, and the first place to search for the cause is in your home. Look for any damp or musty areas, or any condition leading to high humidity, especially if your headaches occur in winter or during the rainy season.

If you accept this premise, you will be on the road to relieving your headaches, and I will do my best to guide you.

The House Dust Mite

Life can be thought of as a series of learning experiences, each of which is filtered through our various cognitive processes until it becomes an essential part of who we are. We may not make use of this knowledge at the time we learn it, but as humans we have the unique ability to store information in our long-term memory banks and to call it forth when we need it.

Much of the new knowledge we acquire is pleasant to recall and fills us with a sense of wonder at the amazing world around us. In some cases, what we learn saddens and even depresses us (like most of what we hear on the six o'clock news each night). And every so often we learn about something that disgusts us or even makes us feel downright squeamish. Well, brace yourself, you're about to acquire some new knowledge in this third category.

I can't think of many things I enjoy discussing less than the house dust mite, except perhaps head lice or body odor. If I could avoid the subject, I would, but I wouldn't be doing right by my patients. The average person who comes to my office has personal hygiene habits that are typical of our modern western culture—I'm sure they shower or bathe regularly, wash their hair at least three times a week, and keep their homes clean and tidy. The last thing they want to be told is that they are sharing their residences with a bunch of creepy little insects. However, the subject is so important that it has to be discussed and at enough length so that people with headaches can understand mites and learn to deal with them effectively.

I'm sure you're probably saying to yourself, "House dust mites? No way, José—I've never seen any in *my* house! Regrettably, you would be wrong. They are in your house. But you would be partially right—you've never seen them—not unless you've been down on your hands and knees lately examining your carpet with a microscope.

The Microscope

If you did look at your carpet with a microscope, you would behold a miniature world populated by these microscopic insects, with their hunched backs and their eight tiny legs, scampering among the carpet fibers like minute campers playing hide and seek among the trees. In some carpets, only a few scurry in and out among the fibers, lonely little critters with few playmates. In other carpets, millions of them crawl contentedly across the miniature landscape.

Whether few or many, they are not possessed of good manners. When nature calls, they relieve their bowels right where they stand, and it is these unappetizing little mite droppings that are important for those who suffer headaches to be aware of.

Scientists have found that many patients react dramatically to the house dust mite. In searching for the reason for this marked reaction, they discovered that this tiny insect carries a potent allergen. (An allergen is the molecule of ragweed, mite, etc., that causes an allergic reaction.) This allergen is most heavily concentrated in the mite droppings.

You may be saying to yourself, "I've heard enough—is there anyplace in the world where there are no mites?" Unfortunately, there is no such place—they live everywhere. Scientists have searched for them in Europe, Asia, South America, North America, Australia, Hawaii, and Africa, and in each of these separate lands, this annoying little bug lives in the everyday dust that collects in the houses.

I guess you could say the house dust mite fits in the same category as death and taxes—they are an unavoidable fact of life. No matter how much we'd like to rid our homes of these creatures, we cannot. However, although we must live with them, there are ways to significantly reduce their growth and numbers. We do this by increasing the problems they face as they try to establish homes within our homes.

What Conditions Encourage the Growth of Mites?

House dust mites are surprisingly similar to humans in their requirements for growth—that's why they get along so well in our environment. Their physical needs are satisfied by the same creature comforts that sustain us so well.

However, there is much debate in the scientific community about whether their emotional needs are being met. Obviously, it is difficult to provide the love and attention so necessary for a pet's well-being through a microscope, and so far, no one has been able to learn their language. However, there are encouraging developments. A large, multicenter study, funded by the government, is exploring ways to communicate with mites.

Arlen C. Jeffers, M.D., Ph.D., of Chalmers Medical School, is particularly enthusiastic about the results of his studies. He has established a primitive sign language to communicate with mites by teaching them to tap a leg in response to his voice—since mites have so many legs, this seems an appropriate approach. He has detected an intellectual ability in the mite equal to that of the typical allergist and believes that, with proper training, it may even surpass them in intelligence.

However hopeful these studies seem, at present there is no way for those who wish to grow mites to provide for their emotional needs. They can only satisfy their physical needs, which include shelter, warmth, food, and moisture. In the following paragraphs, I will discuss these physical needs in more depth (and more seriously, I promise; as you must have guessed by now, there is no Dr. Arlen Jeffers, nor is there a Chalmers Medical School).

Shelter

In days of old, mites had a lot of trouble finding a home. At first there were only dirt, wood, or stone floors in houses, and these provided none of the conditions mites needed to live comfortably.

Then along came the marvelous carpet, with lots of space for mites to frolic in, raise their young, and establish communities—a near-perfect environment but for one repetitive and disastrous event. Every once in awhile, some inconsiderate human would hang the carpet on a clothesline and attack it with a carpet beater. Not only did the beating send uncle, aunt, and cousin mites sailing into the wind, it also disposed of those previously deceased plus a good share of the droppings.

Back then, finding secure housing was truly discouraging for any house dust mite wanting to raise a family. However, their lot has improved dramatically. Through the miracle of modern technology, most homes now contain the perfect shelters for mites. They are called wall-to-wall carpets, permanently installed.

Acres of room to live in (from a mite's perspective) and no way to hang the carpet on a line for anyone to beat it.

The only time of danger for the mite is when its host breaks out the vacuum cleaner (which cleans the surface), but luckily for the mites, this machine has a built-in early warning device, giving them time to scurry to the bottom of the fibers for safety. Aaah, heaven on earth!

Over the years, the same progress has been made in furniture. In the past, chairs were made of wood with no luxurious padding—hardly a fit home for any self-respecting mite. To these microscopic citizens of our homes, living on a wooden chair was like living on a dried-up old lake bed hundreds of miles long and wide. No shelter, no protection. To make the situation even more intolerable, some inconsiderate human would come along and oil the wood, turning the mite's home into a grease pit. Yuck!

Once again, progress rushed to the mite's aid—thickly upholstered armchairs, recliners, and sofas made possible by human ingenuity. Now the mites, along with all of their brothers, sisters, aunts, uncles, cousins, and children, can sleep contentedly at night, secure in their well-stuffed homes.

Bedding is another story of the mite's struggle against adversity. Back when so little shelter was available, mattresses and pillows provided about the only desirable housing for the mite. They're still pretty attractive today, especially if the pillow is stuffed with feathers.

Blankets and sheets used to be washed in boiling hot water, which not only cleaned the bedclothes but went a long way toward filling up the mite cemeteries. It's tough to survive a bath in boiling water! Fortunately, the discovery of cool-water detergents now means a refreshing wash and shampoo for the mite instead of instant death.

Were there a person who, for some peculiar reason, wanted to provide the best environment for this microscopic insect, they could hardly improve on what the modern home already has to offer.

Warmth

Just as we need a warm home to survive winter's chilly temperatures, mites also need warmth to survive—seventy degrees Fahrenheit or above. They share our dread of that horrible day when the furnace fails. However, mites differ from us in their inability to protect themselves against cold—no one has ever observed one wearing a winter coat (at least I haven't run into this observation in any of the medical literature). Besides, they wouldn't know whether to buy gloves or boots for all those feet, and the cost would be prohibitive once you added in the sales tax.

In our grandparents' time, a mite's life in the winter was no bed of roses. The only warmth was found around the pot-bellied stove, and any shelter that existed was strictly second rate. Only that well-beaten carpet laying on a cold floor. The wooden furniture was hardly better than no home at all, and the lightly stuffed furniture only had room for a small mite family, maybe with grandparents. The mattresses and pillows were cold as a devil's heart, and the heated stones that warmed the children's feet were a mite too hot for the little critters—a hazardous situation that few of them survived.

However, modern technology again rushed to the rescue. Today our winterized homes provide a welcome haven for the mite from attic to basement. No more does the mite have to worry about mittens, boots, and warming stones. Its only concern is avoiding heat prostration.

Food

Although finding shelter and warmth has been difficult for the mite until recently, they have always had a ready supply of food. Not being a gourmet diner, I am hesitant to criticize the mite's taste in food, but I know I have no interest in eating at his table. The mite feeds on the skin scales, or dander, we humans shed, and, take my word for it, we shed an unbelievable amount of dander. I recall once seeing a photograph of a man standing in a special light that dramatically showed the amount of dander he was shedding. He looked like a man-shaped lawn sprinkler, spraying dander in all directions. My yard should be watered that well.

We humans will shed dander for as long as our species survives, because the alternative is unacceptable—going through life covered with layers of scaly, dead skin. Would that our food supply were are secure as the dust mite's.

Moisture

As inviting as the shelter, warmth, and food make our modern homes for these microscopic pests, alas, into each life a little rain must fall. Actually, a little rain would solve the mite's problem. It cannot live without moisture. Mites die when the humidity falls below forty to fifty percent. For these helpless creatures, a house where the winter thermometer registers the same temperature found in the kitchen freezer is a frightening place indeed. The cold air is much too dry. Fortunately for allergic humans, the lack of moisture keeps the mite population from reaching its maximum potential in health and numbers.

But there is a place where moisture can be maintained in the home—a place where the mite can flourish. It simply needs air with enough humidity to prevent it from drying out. The one area of your house that is humid both summer and winter is the basement.

Basement moisture is such an important topic for the allergic patient that we will cover it in more detail later, along with other problem areas of the house. But first, we will look at other microscopic house guests that bring pain and discomfort to those who suffer allergic headaches—mold, yeast, and algae.

A Caution to the Reader

By now, I'm sure you know more than you ever cared to about the house dust mite. But as distressing as it is to read about this unappealing insect, it is important for you to have this information because the mite is a predominant cause of allergy.

Many studies point to it as a major culprit in allergic asthma, and it ranks high on the list of allergens that cause chronic nasal blockage. It also contributes mightily to chronic skin itching. My nurses and I find that it is a major cause of headache.

I have tried to soften this information by presenting it with a few chuckles, but any humor you find in this chapter shouldn't lead you to believe the mite is not important. It is.

Make no mistake about the mite. It's presence in your home is no laughing matter, and you must take any measures available to you to reduce its numbers and lessen its impact on your life. I hope to teach you how to do this in a later chapter.

Mold, Yeast, and Algae

We examined the house dust mite because, to understand the genesis of allergic headaches, it is important to understand the role of this microscopic creature with which we share our lives. But it does not live alone in the mite-sheltering areas of the home—the carpets, stuffed furniture, and mattresses. As the flowers in a garden of mixed blossoms are surrounded by other plants, the mite lives in a world populated by other tiny life forms invisible to the naked eye. Viewed through a microscope, this miniature world truly resembles a colorful garden.

The floor of this garden is covered by the roots (hyphae) of growing mold, and the blossoms (mold spores) rise above these roots in a bewildering variety of shapes. Aspergillus mold spreads a clump of spores with the symmetrical shape of a chrysanthemum. Penicillium mold raises clusters of spores that open like daisies, while alternaria spores resemble no known flower, but look more like grotesque war clubs attached handle to end. Other varieties of mold show off their spores in a multitude of sizes and shapes.

Instead of being well-ordered and neat, the mold garden is disordered and messy. Mingled with the plant-like molds are other microscopic life forms whose connected cells resemble chains thrown helter-skelter among the fibers of our carpets and furniture. There are even creatures made up of one cell, actively reproducing by budding off new cells or splitting into two new and identical entities. These many and varied life forms living among the mold spores are called yeast and algae.

Mold, Yeast, and Algae: Similarities

These tiny organisms have many similarities, some of which are as follows: (1) They live together; (2) they need to reproduce and spread; (3) they share the same growth requirements; (4) the same actions discourage their growth.

THEY LIVE TOGETHER. Wherever conditions are suitable for the growth of any one of these three microorganisms, they are suitable for all three. Therefore, the air in a musty basement contains not only mold but also yeast and algae. All three are found in the discharge of a humidifier or the air that rushes from the cushions of an old couch whenever someone sits on it.

THEY NEED TO REPRODUCE AND SPREAD. Mold, yeast, and algae share with all creatures the drive to multiply and spread to new living areas. This means they must "jump" from the carpet to the couch or from the mattress to the book to establish new homes. Whether they make this jump solo or by hitching a ride on a speck of house dust, for awhile they are airborne and can be inhaled by the inhabitants of the house. If they are inhaled by someone who is susceptible to allergic headaches, pain results.

THEY SHARE THE SAME GROWTH REQUIREMENTS. Mold, yeast, and algae share the same need for warmth, food, shelter, and moisture. Wherever excess moisture exists, one is sure to find mold, yeast, and algae.

THE SAME ACTIONS DISCOURAGE THEIR GROWTH. Since they share the same growth requirements, any action by the homeowner that discourages the growth of mold, yeast, and algae will inhibit the ability of all three to multiply and spread.

In practicality, this means that by reducing excess humidity in the home and removing carpets and stuffed furniture from moist areas, the homeowner can reduce the mold, yeast, and algae in the air the headache sufferer must breathe.

Because of these similarities, it is convenient, although somewhat inaccurate, to refer to all three microorganisms—mold, yeast, and algae—as mold. Therefore, although we are discussing each of them individually in this chapter, the term mold will also mean yeast and algae in all other chapters of this book.

Mold, Yeast, and Algae: Differences

Although the person with headaches should regard mold, yeast, and algae as essentially the same, allergists do not. Certain differences are troublesome for doctors who treat allergic illnesses, and these are as follows: (1) There are many different types of molds, yeasts, and algae; (2) only a limited number can be used for testing and treatment.

THERE ARE MANY DIFFERENT TYPES OF MOLDS, YEASTS, AND ALGAE. Cultures of the air inside and outside the home yield a large variety of molds, yeasts, and algae growing on the culture medium. Any one or all of them may cause symptoms for the allergic patient who breathes the air in which they float.

To the immune system, each type of organism is separate and distinct and each has antibodies and lymphocytes committed to fighting them. We will discuss allergy injections in more detail later, but it is sufficient here to mention one of their requirements.

If we want the injection to fight mold, yeast, and algae, it must contain material made from these organisms. This requirement raises questions. Do injections against one type of mold also protect against other types? Do they also protect against yeast and algae? Do mold, yeast, and algae each need to be included in the injections to give patients the protection they deserve? These questions are still not fully answered.

ONLY A LIMITED NUMBER CAN BE USED FOR TESTING OR TREATMENT. In general, to test or treat patients with injections of molds, yeasts, and algae, they must first be grown in the laboratory of pharmaceutical companies that manufacture these solutions. Many will not grow in the laboratory. Perhaps the best illustration are the mushrooms to which many people react with sneezing, wheezing, and other symptoms. They grow poorly in the lab.

Even if tests could be prepared for these hundreds of different organisms, it would be impractical and much too costly to test for each one. Similarly, treatment using these huge numbers of different organisms would be impossible, as there far are too many.

Does this mean that treatment of allergies due to mold, yeast, and algae is impossible? No, not at all. In our practice, we find that including a representative number of these organisms in our allergy injection treatment provides much headache relief for our patients.

Research continues to expand our knowledge of allergic illness caused by the microscopic organisms that fill the air we breathe. Although I look forward to the benefits of future research, I also am grateful for the past research that has given me such powerful therapies with which to treat my patients with allergy.

Making Mold, Yeast, and Algae Unwelcome in Your Home

Treatment with allergy injections provides marvelous headache relief to the allergic patient, but an even better way of gaining relief is simply avoidance. If those who are sensitive to mold, yeast, and algae can avoid excessive exposure to these microorganisms, they can prevent the debilitating symptoms they cause.

How can this be done? By following the same advice I gave when we discussed the house dust mite. Because yeast, mold, and algae share the mite's need for moisture and shelter, making the home inhospitable to mites also makes it inhospitable to these pesky microorganisms.

* * *

Many people worry about the yeast and mold found in foods. In many cases, their concern is appropriate, but they do not realize that they are ignoring another potent exposure to these organisms. The air in their basements may be loaded with yeast and mold, and as they breathe, some is absorbed through the nose and lungs and some through the intestine from swallowing nasal drainage. In effect, they are "eating" mold and yeast with every breath they take.

If these people want to reduce the mold and yeast they consume, they should look for and eliminate problems that produce mold and yeast in the air in their homes. We will examine ways to do that next.

Part III
Correcting Excessive Moisture, Mites, and Mold

Combatting Moisture

To control either your own headaches or those of a loved one, you will need to reduce the excess moisture in your home that breeds house dust mites, mold, yeast, and algae. Dryness is their nemesis, an archenemy they cannot survive. It is the key to reaching the precious goal of days free from pain.

To help you reach this goal, in the following chapters, I will present some recommendations for combatting moisture problems. But before I do that, I want to clarify a few points and caution you about at least one thing. I also want to remind you that, as mentioned in the previous chapter, to avoid repetition of the terms mold, yeast, and algae, I will refer to all three as mold because wherever one is found, all three are present.

Some Clarifications

By moisture, I do not mean standing water or water running across the floor. You do not need to have puddles of water in your basement to produce the moisture necessary for mite and mold growth. Nor is it necessary to have steam bath levels of humidity—the amount of humidity found in the typical "dry" basement is more than adequate.

In the average home, there are many areas where moisture is present in sufficient quantities to sustain dust mites and mold. We will discuss all of them; however, we will spend a fair amount of time examining the basement, because it is there that humidity is most consistently present and most persistent.

It is not necessary to kill off all the dust mites and mold in the home. That would be impossible. Rendering the air completely free of them would be no less a task than emptying the ocean by throwing seawater up on the shore, and only the uninformed would attempt it. Even if it were possible, dust mites and mold exist everywhere, both inside and outside the home, and as quickly as the water would run from the shore back into the sea, they would flood back into the home.

Fortunately, it is not necessary to completely eliminate them. Even the most sensitive headache sufferer can tolerate low levels of both. Our task is to aggressively attack and correct conditions that lead to excessive growth of these organisms. That's how we stop headaches.

Although both the home and the workplace can have high enough levels of moisture to grow dust mites and mold, we will concentrate on the home. There are often excessive numbers of these headache-producing microorganisms in the workplace, but the worker usually has little influence over conditions there, and trying to force a change in the work environment can anger employers and threaten job security. We will discuss this in more detail when we examine the occurrence of headaches at work.

On the other hand, in the home, whether owned or rented, the occupant can exercise more control and can choose to make conditions dryer. These dryer conditions, low in dust mites and mold, can mean such improvement in symptoms that the headache sufferer becomes more resistant to these aggravating pains both at home and in the workplace. I have seen this happen on many occasions.

A realistic timetable is perfectly acceptable. Many of the actions I will recommend are easy and inexpensive—you can do them right away. Others will be expensive (removing a basement carpet) or emotionally wrenching (getting rid of your favorite plants or your treasured collection of books), and you will have to plan when and how to accomplish them. That's fine. Do your planning and accomplish the task as soon as you are able.

As a rule of thumb, if my patients can accomplish the hard parts of improving their environment within five years of their first visit to my office, I am satisfied.

Each action you take to improve your environment has a good chance of helping you reduce your headaches. Whether the remedy is difficult or easy, expensive or cheap, emotionally wrenching or not, it should help you feel better. It will be worth the effort.

Accomplish the easy things as quickly as possible and you will soon be repaid for your efforts as you suffer less. Once you have taken care of the easier remedies, if your headaches are reduced to a level you can tolerate, you may find you can take more time to do the more difficult tasks.

A Caution

I am an allergist, and not an expert in designing or constructing homes. The only structure I ever built was a playhouse made of four-by-eight plywood sheets (no child would play in it, which speaks volumes about my construction abilities). Therefore, some of my recommendations may not be realistic, even though I believe in them strongly and want them to be helpful. Please discuss these suggestions with an appropriate specialist in home construction or repair before implementing them.

The reason I present this advice to you is that I believe it to be correct, and during my years of treating patients with headaches, I have found it to be beneficial in controlling their pain. I have also found the opposite to be true: where patients were unable or unwilling to eliminate exposures to moisture or mustiness, our treatment has yielded results that were much less than satisfactory.

Learning About Moisture

My nurses and I have come to realize that treating our patients without inquiring about sources of excess moisture, dust mites, and mold in their homes is like riding a bicycle with a flat tire. It's possible, but why would anyone try it? If we do not uncover these problem areas, and if our patients do not correct them to the maximum extent possible, our treatment will have disappointing results.

Making this inquiry is so important that we launch it on our patients' first visit. Some of the questions we ask are:

- What type of house or apartment do you live in?
- Where is the house situated?
- Does water drain away from the house?
- What is in the basement?
- What is upstairs?

There is good reason for our questions—our treatment will fail if the patient's environment is damp. Allergy treatment is potent and almost always provides our patients good relief from their headaches, but it can be overpowered by a poor environment. The moist home is like the thousand-pound gorilla that crashes the dinner party—get rid of it or no dinner party.

To get rid of the gorilla—to eliminate the moisture—you must know where to find it and what to do about it. The next few chapters will look at unfavorable conditions in the home in more detail and recommend ways for the homeowner to remedy these conditions. I have presented some general information on moisture problems in earlier chapters, but examining it in more specific terms will provide you with knowledge that can make life more comfortable.

The Concrete Slab in Contact with the Ground

When a famous bank robber was asked why he robbed banks, he replied something like this: "Because that's where the money is." While I may not admire his career choice, I have to admit he showed great practicality in going directly to the number one source of money. Let's follow his lead and go directly to the number one source of moisture in our homes—the concrete slab on which it rests.

It is a common misconception that most of the moisture in our basements enters through the walls. After all, they are the most obvious source, and our attention is certainly focused on them during periods of heavy rain or when the ground is saturated with water.

My patients with headaches share this misconception and often resist the idea that their basement could be damp, offering such proofs of dryness as: "I have a walkout basement," or "My basement has three big windows," or "Two (or three) sides of my basement are above ground."

If you focus only on the walls of your basement, you can be misled the same way an unwary home buyer is deceived by the fresh coat of paint covering a crumbling exterior. By concentrating on the walls (and on whether or not they are above or below ground), you will fail to recognize the importance of the concrete slab beneath your feet.

Why is the slab so important? To me, it's what makes a particular area a basement. Indeed, my definition of a basement (at least, for the allergic person) is any area with a concrete slab in contact with the underlying soil. This definition does not change even when all four walls of a structure are entirely above ground but the slab is laid directly on the ground, which is standard construction practice in some places.

Why is the concrete slab so worrisome? Because, in reality, it is nothing more than a dirt floor. This may surprise you since it is so nice and level, is usually a pleasant whitish-gray in color, and can be swept clean with a broom. These characteristics make it similar to a wood floor, but unlike wood, a concrete floor is composed of sand, gravel, and cement—materials extracted from the soil.

Being made of cement, sand, and gravel give the concrete floor one important characteristic that makes it different from floors made of other materials. The sand and gravel mixture makes it porous, and this makes it possible for moisture to rise from the underlying soil to the surface of the slab the way a candle's wick allows melted wax to rise to the flame.

Once the moisture "wicks" its way to the surface, it evaporates into the air, where it becomes the humidity that is usually present in your basement. This humidity is often high enough to ensure the abundant growth of house dust mites and mold.

Neither of these pesky problems requires standing water, but both need a relative humidity of forty percent or higher. Without it they die. The moisture rising from the basement floor ensures them this life-sustaining humidity level and often causes humidity levels that are high enough for dust mites and mold to grow abundantly. As long as conditions exist that allow them to thrive, these unwanted guests will stimulate the headaches that plague my patients.

Obviously, any action that reduces this humidity is an action that will prevent headaches. It should be equally obvious that reducing the moisture arising from the cement slab is an excellent way to reduce humidity.

We will discuss some things you can do to lower the humidity level in your basement, but first we should look at some actions you can take outside your home, actions that will dry out the soil under the slab and thus reduce the amount of moisture that seeps through it. Let's see how this can be done.

Moisture in the Soil Beneath the Slab

Ever backed up and tripped over something, falling and landing on that part of your anatomy my grandmother referred to as your "caboose"? (My grandfather was a railroad engineer, so Grandmother adopted railroad terms for lots of things.) I know I have, many times.

What if you landed in a puddle? I've done that, too. When this happened, didn't you wish you had fallen on dry ground? It wasn't bad enough you had to suffer the embarrassment of taking a spill, not to mention a possible injury to your tailbone, but remember what it felt like to end up with a wet "sitter," too?

Well, if your house were capable of sensation, you can well imagine how it would feel having to sit in wet ground all the time. This example will help you understand how the wetness saturates the concrete slab resting on it and allows moisture to penetrate it.

Clearly, the way to prevent this is to build on dry ground, and there are ways to check soil moisture before a house is built. But short of drilling holes in the basement floor, there is no way to know for sure how much moisture is in the soil beneath an existing structure. However, there are some clues that will help you determine whether you have a soil moisture problem:

- Is the house located near a stream, pond, or swamp? If so, the ground is probably wet.

- Is it near a lake, and if so, is it on the level of the lake or on a hill above it? The air blowing over a lake is likely to be more humid than air blowing over dry land, and the soil at lake level is more likely to be wet than the soil on a hill above a lake.

- Is the soil clay or sand? Clay drains water poorly, and building a house on clay is like building it in a bathtub without a drain.

- Do the neighbors need a sump pump to keep their basements from flooding? A sump pump is good evidence the soil does not drain well.

- Is the house located in a wooded area or on a prairie? A prairie should have dry ground on which to build a home plus good ventilating breezes to blow away moisture.

The answers to these questions are good indicators of the water content of the soil. We ask them of our new patients, and you would do well to keep them in mind when evaluating your present house or searching for a new one. They will help you determine whether a house rests in damp soil.

Unfortunately, even the correct answers to these questions won't guarantee that the home you build or buy will be dry. For instance, you may think that sandy soil guarantees a dry house. This may not be true—in some cases, sandy soils drain poorly because an impervious layer of clay beneath the sand traps water under the house and prevents it from draining away. Despite indications to the contrary, the basement may be wet.

To further complicate matters, seemingly dry land may have an underground spring nearby that saturates the soil and makes the basement humid. Furthermore, even sandy soil with good drainage is never completely dry. It always has some ground moisture that transmits to the slab. Thus, even apparently dry land may contain headache-causing moisture.

The opposite may also be true. Houses in apparently went soil can be relatively dry. My home rests in a "bath-tub" of clay soil, and many of the neighboring homes require sump pumps. Yet our house does not need a pump. I can't explain why this is so.

What Can You Do?

As you probably realize by now, there is no way to guarantee that the soil beneath the cement slab of an existing home is dry. Also, there is no way to guarantee that if the soil is dry when a house is built, it will remain so throughout its lifetime. (A neighbor's previously dry basement flooded when nearby home construction changed the surrounding landscape drainage.)

Although land is never perfectly dry, the person with headaches should not give up trying to find a home that is as dry as possible. Avoid purchasing land near lakes, ponds, streams, and swamps. If possible, take soil samples. Have the contractor add adequate drainage systems to carry away water that may collect under the concrete slab.

Use the same precautions when buying an existing home. Select one that is located where the land is more likely than not to be dry. Pass up the home that presents a risk of soil moisture, even though it may be less expensive. A bargain home built on wet soil is a poor investment—what you save on the price of the home may be spent on treating chronic headaches.

Above all else, even if your land is dry, always assume there is some dampness in the soil and that the cement slab is bringing excess moisture into the basement. We will discuss ways to combat this moisture, the first and most important of which is to ensure that the home has proper landscape drainage, which is the subject of the next chapter.

Landscape Drainage

The importance of properly draining rainwater away from your house cannot be overemphasized. How pointless it is to build a house on dry soil if rainwater and snow melt is allowed to collect at its foundation, wetting the soil around the basement walls and beneath the concrete slab? All the homeowner's fine planning is for naught. The basement will support a huge population of house dust mites and mold. The allergic occupant's headaches will be multiple and miserable.

This need not be so. There are ways to make sure that water drains away from your house. First, watch what happens to the water after it falls on the roof, flows into the gutters and through the downspouts, and then spills onto the ground. Is this collection system intact and properly placed? Does the downspout deposit the water into an area that will carry it away from the house? Second, correct any problems you spot. It's that simple (at least it sounds that simple to me).

If your house lacks gutters, or if the gutters leak or are clogged with leaves and other debris, the water will pour onto the ground beside the house, wetting the basement walls and floor. Install new gutters or repair and clean out the existing ones so that water from the roof is carried to the downspouts. Then watch the water as it flows from the downspouts into the yard. If it collects near the foundation, change the direction of the downspouts to an area with good drainage. If that doesn't work, consult an expert for suggestions or consider moving.

My own experience convinces me that this advice works. As I mentioned in a previous chapter, the direction of one of my downspouts had to be changed so the water it carried would flow down a nearby hill instead of soaking under my garage. What I did not mention is another problem that had to be solved earlier.

My house rests in clay soil, and rainwater frequently seeped into the basement, running across the floor until it escaped through a floor drain. When it rained, my basement took on the fragrance of a swamp. I discovered that a downspout on the side of the house opposite from the one mentioned above emptied onto level ground, allowing the water to pool near the foundation, where it soaked into the soil. Once the soil was saturated, water leaked into the basement.

In surveying my yard, I found there was no nearby downward slope where this water could be directed. The closest one was thirty feet away, and a small hill blocked access to it. I had to dig a trench through the top of this hill to gain access to this downslope. Once this project was finished, the rainwater was able to drain away from the house and lost all interest in leaking into my basement. There was a noticeable improvement in how it smelled.

Now it requires an extremely heavy rain to send even a small trickle of water onto the basement floor, and this is not a catastrophe. The floor is bare and the water is easily mopped up. Because my basement walls and slab are now dry, house dust mites and mold no longer flourish in my home.

Check your landscape drainage. Put on a raincoat, grab an umbrella, and venture outside on a rainy day if there is no lightning. Watch what happens to the rainwater after it falls on your roof. Does it drain away properly? Does water from the neighboring areas flow toward your house? If you see a problem, correct it or hire a professional to correct it.

Good landscape drainage is overwhelmingly important. It will help keep your soil dry and reduce the amount of moisture that penetrates the concrete slab. Your basement will be less humid, and fewer numbers of dust mites and mold will grow there. You will suffer far fewer headaches.

Ensuring a dry slab is essential to maintaining a dry home, but other actions should also be pursued. We will explore these further remedies as we continue to examine conditions in the home that lead to headaches.

Basement Bedrooms and Offices

The basement is not a friendly place for the person who suffers headaches. As we discussed earlier, too much moisture escapes from the concrete slab, elevating the humidity and prompting the growth of house dust mites and mold, two major causes of headaches.

Whether homeowners finish their basements, what rooms they build there, how they furnish these rooms, and how much time they spend there will have a major impact on the number and severity of the headaches they suffer. These factors can spell the difference between mildly irritating pain and incapacitating agony. For this reason, the time we spend considering this important area is not wasted.

Let's examine the rooms that may be constructed in the basement and discuss ways to minimize the problems this creates.

The Basement Bedroom

A bedroom contains many shelters for mites and mold. Carpets, books, and overstuffed furniture—found in any room of the house—plus mattresses and bedding, found only in the bedroom, provide luxurious places for these nuisances to thrive.

Not only is the shelter excellent, the high-humidity environment of a bedroom with a concrete floor encourages mites and mold to multiply rapidly. The headache sufferer sleeping in this room should not be surprised if they have frequent and distressing pain. What a terrible place for them to sleep!

My staff and I know we must identify those patients who sleep in the basement and persuade them to move to an upstairs bedroom. The importance of this advice cannot be overemphasized. Of all our patients, those who sleep in the basement suffer the most frequent and painful sinus and migraine headaches. Moving out of the basement bedroom almost always reduces these headaches, making the inconvenience worthwhile.

Although it is imperative for the headache sufferer to leave, it is sometimes impossible. For instance, a large family living in a small house may need the extra bedroom space found only in the basement. In cases where the house was originally constructed with all the bedrooms in the basement, the arrangement cannot be changed.

If the patient with headaches must remain in a basement bedroom, great care must be taken to diminish its humidity and reduce the numbers of dust mites and mold found there. The following are helpful suggestions:

- Wash the blankets and sheets frequently in hot, soapy water.

- Encase the mattress and box spring in zip-up plastic covers.

- Store few or no books in the basement.

- Ensure adequate ventilation to keep the room as dry as possible.

- Use a dehumidifier from spring through fall.

- Use furniture with little or no stuffing.

- Tile the floor and use small throw rugs that can be easily cleaned.

Mary Beth's Story

These measures, although not as effective as moving to an upstairs bedroom, can help reduce headaches tremendously. I remember vividly what happened to Mary Beth, a young lady whose headaches (plus other allergic illnesses) were awful in spite of her undergoing allergy injections and making many dietary changes. They were so severe that she had consulted neurologists on many occasions, had undergone elaborate and expensive tests, and had visited the emergency room on a number of occasions when her headache pain became overwhelming.

She eventually overcame these terrible headaches, but the story of how she did it was surprising. As she told me about it, our conversation went something like this. I was asking her the usual questions about her headaches when she said, "Dr. Walsh, you have been telling me for two years that I need to move from my basement bedroom if I want to get my headaches under better control."

"It really matters, Mary Beth," I replied, wondering where this conversation was leading. I felt she wanted to tell me something, and I hoped she wasn't about to insist again that the bedroom didn't cause her headaches. We had had that disagreement on her last visit.

"I found that out," she replied. "After a week of crushing migraine headaches, I decided out of desperation to follow your suggestions about the bedroom."

"Did you move to an upstairs bedroom?" I asked.

"I couldn't, Dr. Walsh. With three children upstairs, there is no room for me. But three months ago I removed the carpet and pad and covered the mattress in plastic. It worked! Now I can go a week or more without a getting headache."

"I'm so pleased, Mary Beth," I replied—and I was. Prior to making these changes in her bedroom, in spite of our treatment, she had never had a week without frequent—often daily—headaches.

"I became even more convinced that the bedroom was a major cause of my headaches after a peculiar thing happened," she said. "I decided that, since encasing the mattress in plastic helped so much, I would do the same thing with the box spring. As I was struggling with it, I suddenly got sick. My eyes swelled, I started wheezing and couldn't catch my breath, and I ended up with one of the worst headaches of my whole life."

Mary Beth was amazed that the dust stirred up just by handling the box spring brought on such overwhelming and painful symptoms. I was also surprised. Although I am convinced that sleeping in the basement causes headaches, a story like Mary Beth's, providing such dramatic confirmation of the headache-producing potency of this exposure, is shocking. No wonder that, years after it happened, it sticks in my memory.

Stories similar to how Mary Beth's allergy reacted to mites and mold in her mattress and box spring have been told to me repeatedly by other patients. They are strong evidence of the pain-provoking power of the basement bedroom.

If at all possible, avoid having a bedroom in the basement. If you must sleep there, however, do as Mary Beth did and follow the steps I listed above.

The Basement Office or Work Area

The same problems that affect the basement bedroom pervade the basement office or work area. Carpeting, stuffed furniture, and books harbor mites and mold, and the person working in this area is exposed to higher concentrations of these organisms than in any other part of the house. Add to that the large amount of paper that is used and stored in an office and the exposure becomes even worse. Our allergic patients who use these areas are plagued by frequent and painful headaches. If it is possible to move the office or work area to the first or second floor, do so. Your head will be grateful.

Many of our patients find this move impossible, however. In some cases, they run businesses out of their home that demand so much work area, only the basement is suitable. One of my patients is a seamstress whose sewing machines and cutting area occupy a large amount of space. I also treat a husband and wife team that has a computer operation in the basement and another couple that runs an accounting business from a basement office.

Several of my patients groom dogs in their homes, and of course they do so in the only area where such an activity is practical—the basement. (An allergic person who works as a dog groomer is like a diabetic employed as a candy taster or an alcoholic employed as a wine taster—they would be a lot better off if they had chosen another occupation.) When I think of the conditions that must exist in these work areas, I sometimes wonder whether the dust mite and mold levels should be measured not by the gram but by the pound.

If you must work in your basement, follow the same precautions you would with a basement bedroom. To the extent possible, eliminate carpets, stuffed furniture, and any books or papers not absolutely necessary to operating your business. When conditions permit, move your office upstairs or completely out of the home.

The basement is a poor place for the headache sufferer to sleep or work.

Home Age and Construction

The age and the type of home are factors that have a major impact on my patients' headaches. This became very apparent to me soon after I entered practice and started seeing an increasing number of patients who complained of miserable head pain.

Why were they suffering? What factors distinguish them from people free of headaches? Slowly the answers to these questions emerged, and some of these answers pointed to my patients' homes. Certain homes seem to spawn headaches, and my patients must understand their characteristics so they can avoid these characteristics when purchasing or renting a home or change them in their existing home. Two of the most important characteristics are the age of the dwelling and the way it is constructed.

The Older Home—Ellie's Story

Among my patients, those who suffer the most tend to live in the oldest homes. Maybe this is to be expected. Along with memories, perhaps another, not-so-pleasant legacy of the passing years is increased house dust mites and mold in the wood, insulation, and basements.

Many patients living in older dwellings relate tales of headaches that are pitiable. Ellie was one of these patients. I treated her years ago, but I remember her story vividly today.

A fifty-five-year-old homemaker and mother of five teenage boys, Ellie was sent to me by her family doctor when her daily migraine headaches refused to respond to medication. She had already consulted a neurologist (the neurological exam showed no cause for the headaches) and had had elaborate studies done, including special x-rays (these were also normal).

Ellie lived in a ninety-year-old home that had a basement with a dirt floor. Not only was the basement damp smelling in the rainy seasons of spring and fall, but this dampness had permeated the house over those ninety years. When Ellie told me about her home, I was discouraged. Could I provide her with effective treatment while she lived in such an environment?

At my urging, she emptied the basement of everything that could harbor mites and mold, including furniture stored there for the children when they married. She covered the floor with plastic to retard the passage of moisture from the dirt into the air of the basement. She also bought a dehumidifier and began using it regularly.

Although at first I was doubtful that our treatment would help, I was later delighted to learn that her headaches were dwindling. A combination of environmental changes, medications, diet changes, and injections reduced the frequency of her migraines from daily to weekly and took away much of their horrendous pain. Ellie was grateful for the relief.

She was even happier when I saw her some years later. When her husband retired and the children moved out, they sold the old house and moved to a third-floor apartment in a newer building. Her migraines disappeared; she needed no more treatment.

Ellie's story is powerful evidence of the older home's propensity to cause headaches (plus asthma and many other allergic illnesses). If you have headaches and are living in an old house, do what she did. Empty the basement—remove any shelter for mites and mold—and dehumidify it. Preferably the floor is not made of dirt, but if it is, cover it with plastic. Avoid spending time there. Move to a better environment as soon as you can.

Not every older house is musty. Many venerable old structures are free of mustiness and are not apt to cause headaches. In some cases, older houses that are musty can be dried out using dehumidifying, landscape drainage, and the other remedies we discussed. If you must live in an older home, do everything you can to dry it out and to keep it dry.

The Split-Level or Split-Entry Home

In recent years, one of the most popular home construction styles has been the split-level or split-entry style. Unfortunately for the allergic person, this type of home is a poor place to live. In these homes, the floor in some of the living areas is a concrete slab resting on moist soil.

Any area of the home with a concrete floor resting on the ground is a basement and subject to the same excess moisture, mites, and mold conditions. Because of the concrete floor, the humidity will probably be higher than in living areas that have a wood floor. Mites and mold will find ample shelter in which to grow and prosper in the carpet, stuffed furniture, books, and other items in this overly humid area.

To deny shelter to these microorganisms, I advise my patients to cover the cement with tile instead of permanently attached carpeting and to use small area rugs that can be cleaned or replaced. Avoid having stuffed furniture or books in these areas, and don't use them for storage. Most importantly, do not use them for bedrooms if at all possible.

Don't provide shelter for mites and mold in rooms that rest on concrete.

The Home with a Crawl Space

Patients often ask me if purchasing a home with a crawl space is better than buying one with a basement. I don't think so. In fact, I suspect that a crawl space might breed more moisture, dust mites, and mold than a conventional basement.

I believe the home with a basement has an important advantage over the home with a crawl space. The basement can easily be inspected for evidence of damage and water leakage. How often would the crawl space be examined? If the homeowner shared my fear of small, enclosed spaces, the inspections would be few and far between, allowing water and mold problems to develop without being noticed and corrected.

The crawl space is a miniature basement requiring the same air circulation and dehumidifying that is far easier to accomplish in a regular basement. In many homes, the crawl space is not vented to the outside to flush out stale air. Instead, it either is not vented at all or is vented into the basement, producing in this area conditions that encourage the moisture, mite, and mold growth we work so hard to defeat. I also suspect that the moist air of the crawl space infiltrates into the room above it.

If you can avoid having a crawl space in your home, do so. If you have one, consider doing the following:

- Cover the floor of the crawl space with plastic to retard the movement of soil moisture into the area.

- Insulate the ceiling of the crawl space and install a vapor barrier to retard the passage of air from the crawl space into the home.

- Try to vent the crawl space air to the outside. You may need expert advice and help on this project.

As you might have surmised from the above discussion, I am very concerned about crawl spaces.

The Home with a Partitioned Basement

As though it weren't bad enough that we humans behave like pack rats, hoarding things and storing them in our basements, we also imitate beavers in our need to build things down there. Show a man an empty basement and he develops an irresistible urge to grab hammer and saw. He attaches paneling to the cinder block. He erects walls to partition off bedrooms, offices, and family rooms. Then he paints the walls, stands back to admire them, and thinks to himself, "Aren't I smart?" Unfortunately, if a member of his family is allergic, the answer is no.

The reason is that if the basement is left as one large room, it is possible for a dehumidifier to keep the entire area relatively dry. However, separating it into a number of isolated areas severely restricts the movement of moist air to the dehumidifier. The air can't pass through the walls.

Even if heating and cooling ducts are able to keep the air in these rooms dry during the hot summer and cold winter, they do a poor job of reducing the humidity during the spring and fall. Mite and mold growth during these seasons is not likely to be kept in check.

Even worse, I hate to think what might be growing between the cinder block walls and the paneling attached to them. On many occasions, my patients have torn apart these walls and found some nasty surprises.

If you must use the basement for bedrooms or offices, try to keep these areas open so ventilation is not blocked. Try not to panel the walls—paneling covers up any moisture problems, and what is hidden cannot be corrected. Painting the walls with a waterproof paint such as an epoxy is fine.

Better yet, don't build in the basement—remodel the attic or add on to your home if you need more living space. Even better, choose a house with enough space that you are not forced to use the basement.

When we tell our patients that their problems may be due to their finished basement, they frequently reply, "Don't worry, we seldom go down there." (An obvious question comes to mind when I hear this reply: If you don't use the little rooms you built in the basement, why did you build them in the first place?) But they don't need to go down there to breathe the basement air. It migrates to the rest of the house, causing headaches for those who spend both waking and sleeping hours in the living areas above it.

Please consider very carefully any plans to partition your basement into rooms. Think it through at least ten times. Then, don't do it.

The Home Without a Basement or Crawl Space

I recall one day questioning a patient I had been treating for some time whose headaches weren't getting any better. In fact, they were getting worse—much worse.

I was mystified as to why was she was still suffering. She took her dust and mold injections faithfully and avoided the foods and beverages that caused her headaches. "Jane," I asked, "tell me about your house." I suspected that some moisture problem at home was defeating our headache treatment.

"You don't need to worry about my house, Dr. Walsh. It's dry," she replied, knowing that I would be questioning her about moisture in her home. "We moved to a new house six months ago," she told me proudly. "I know you are worried about basement moisture, so we bought a house without a basement."

I was disturbed by Jane's reply. Our questions about the condition of her basement in previous consultations had alerted her to the moisture, mites, and mold found there, and she had resolved not to have a musty basement in her new house. To my chagrin, she had entirely missed the important point that any room with a cement floor in contact with the underlying soil is a basement.

If a house has no basement and the first floor rests on a cement slab, in effect, the first floor becomes the basement. All the carpets, stuffed furniture, books, bedclothing, and other items capable of sheltering mites and mold do so. Both her living room and bedroom were located on the first floor and rested on the concrete slab. I suspected both had high levels of moisture and harbored enough mites and mold to accelerate her headaches. I no longer had any doubt about why she was experiencing so much head pain.

Jane's story concerns me. How many patients misunderstand our questions and advice? The results of studies of doctor–patient communications show that only about one-forth of the information we give our patients is understood; seventy-five percent is lost due to the many distractions in a medical office. I have no trouble believing these findings.

No matter how hard my nurses and I try to educate our patients, there is always a chance for error. My desire to avoid these misunderstandings is a primary factor in my decision to write this book.

Condominiums and town houses are frequently constructed on a concrete slab and lack the buffering space provided by a basement—a space for installing a dehumidifier to interrupt the passage of moisture. If you suffer headaches, avoid these types of homes.

The Home with Poor Ventilation

We who dwell in the northern states have learned to protect ourselves from the hostile winter weather. To keep from freezing in the bitterly cold temperatures and biting winds, we bundle up in layers of clothes until we look like pudgy bears, secure in the warmth of this cosy insulation.

(There's one difference, of course. Bears are smart enough to hibernate during the winter.)

Over the years, we have adopted this same philosophy in our construction practices. To keep our homes warmer and to decrease energy consumption, we add sheathing to the outside, stuff thick layers of insulation between the studs and joists, and then cover everything with a layer of plastic. This layer of plastic serves two important purposes: it keeps out the howling winds and also acts as a moisture barrier to protect the plasterboard on the inside from water damage. But it also has an adverse effect: it keeps your house from breathing.

It may seems ridiculous to think that a house built of wood and cement needs to breathe, but it does. If a house does not exchange its stale air for clean air from the outside, the air breathed by its occupants becomes increasingly foul, not to mention dangerous.

I was reminded of this recently as I reviewed a pamphlet from the American Lung Association entitled "Air Pollution in Your Home." This pamphlet lists the fumes and particles that can be contained in the air of the poorly ventilated house until "air pollution can be much greater inside the home than outside." These fumes and particles and their sources include:

- *Nitrogen dioxide*—from gas appliances, fireplaces, stoves.

- *Carbon monoxide*—from the above sources plus other combustion sources and tobacco smoke.

- *Formaldehyde*—from foam insulation, building materials, carpets, and other materials.

- *Second-hand smoke.*

- *Household products*—cleaners, hobby supplies, etc.

- *Personal care products.*

- *Microbes and fungi.*

A house that is too tightly insulated accumulates fumes from the compounds used to clean the bathroom sink and the kitchen floor as well as from the carpet and the adhesives used in the walls. It collects formaldehyde from manufactured products and smoke from the fireplace. The air we breathe can become worse than the air in the most polluted intersection of the city if it is not allowed to escape and be replaced with fresh air.

Today's tightly constructed homes are also susceptible to another danger—the poorly vented heating system. At least twice a year, I receive a call from a patient with unceasing headaches who tells me that they had their furnace checked and found it was leaking combustion products into the house. Their headaches ceased once the furnace was properly vented. Your furnace may be spewing fumes into your home and you may not know it unless your heating system is inspected by a qualified furnace inspector. I have my furnace checked every year. Because of the danger of asphyxiation, every homeowner should do the same.

Not only does the poorly ventilated home accumulate fumes, it also has high concentrations of moisture. As we breathe, cook, bathe, wash dishes and clothing, mop the floors, and water plants, moisture is released into the air in our homes in the form of humidity. This humidity can cause mold to grow on the window sills and sometimes even in the closets from the basement to the top level of a house. Needless to say, mites and mold find this humidity absolutely wonderful, but people with headaches don't.

Recognizing that a house is poorly ventilated is sometimes difficult. Be suspicious if you notice an especially thick layer of ice on the windows in winter, if your home has a noticeable odor or stuffiness, or if you see mold growing anywhere in the house. Sometimes these clues are absent, but you should suspect poor ventilation if your house is less than fifteen years old (recently built homes tend to be more tightly insulated) and your headaches are frequent, severe, and resistant to treatment.

When our patients respond poorly to treatment, when migraine and sinus headaches persist in spite of weekly allergy injections and good diet control, my staff and I suspect their homes are inadequately ventilated. We also suspect poor ventilation when our patients complain—paradoxically—of sore throats from "dry air." This feeling of dryness occurs because the humidity has allowed mite and mold to reach concentrations that irritate their throats. This irritation causes the sore throat symptoms along with the sensation of dryness.

The poorly ventilated home's propensity to cause illness is acknowledged by the American Lung Association in a pamphlet entitled, "Home Indoor Quality Checklist," which I resurrected from my files. Under the column heading "Strength of Indoor Contaminants," one of the questions listed is:

> Are any of the following symptoms noticeable among residents: headaches, itchy or watery eyes, nose or throat infections or dryness, dizziness, nausea, colds, sinus problems?

To gain relief from the painful headaches caused by inadequate ventilation, your house must be allowed to breathe. Appliances that perform this function are called air exchangers. Best installed during construction, they replace stale air with clean, fresh air from outside the home. They are expensive but potentially will save money that would otherwise be spent on medical bills and lost wages.

Few of my patients have lived in homes with air exchangers long enough for me to know whether these devices completely cure problems with moisture and fumes. However, I believe they should be built into any new, tightly insulated and weatherstripped house and retrofitted into poorly vented older houses.

What if your home is poorly ventilated and you can't afford to install an air exchanger? Leaving a window open throughout the winter might solve the ventilation problem, but the increased energy cost due to heat loss through the window might outweigh the cost of installing an air exchanger.

Further information on the poorly ventilated home is readily available from the library or from units of government. For example, the Minnesota Department of Public Service (790 American Center, 150 E. Kellogg Boulevard, Saint Paul, Minnesota 55101) publishes two pertinent pamphlets: "Home Moisture Problems" and "Combustion Air."

The Living Area or Apartment Built Over a Garage

Many of our patients with frequent and painful headaches live in apartments situated over garages or in homes with tuck-under garages. The likely cause of these increased symptoms is that the leakage of air from the garage into the living spaces brings moisture and fumes into the home.

I am sure not all apartments situated over garages or houses with tuck-under garages share this problem, but my experience treating patients who live in these situations leads me to believe that many do. Often patients tell me they smell an exhaust-like odor in their home or apartment, indicating some communication with the air of the garage. One patient's story was particularly convincing. He described how he carefully sealed the holes in the floor that separates his apartment from the garage and how his headaches improved for years afterward. Unfortunately, his headaches have returned, and I suspect that new openings have developed or his patches no longer prevent air leakage from the garage.

People with headaches should avoid living areas or apartments located above a garage.

The Ground-Level Apartment

The moisture problems that affect people living in areas of the home that have a cement floor resting on the ground also affect those living on the bottom floor of an apartment building. It does not matter whether the bottom floor is at ground level or below the ground, or whether it is called a basement, garden-level, or first-floor apartment. Moisture from the soil penetrates the cement resting on it, escapes into the air of the apartment, and causes unwelcome humidity.

This can be a particularly cruel hardship for many of my patients. Those who live in these apartments usually do so because they have no other choice. In some cases, they are unable to live higher up because age or poor health makes climbing stairs difficult or impossible. In other cases, they can only afford the rent for a lower-level apartment, which is often significantly less. Whether infirm or poor, these patients cannot move, which is a shame.

If possible, patients with headaches should avoid such apartments.

The Mobile Home

Unfortunately, mobile homes are another example of low-cost or accessible housing that does not seem to be acceptable for our patients with headaches. While they may be attractive for those with limited finances, the money saved in housing costs is often wasted on doctor bills, medication, and days lost from work. Unfortunately, people who find themselves in these circumstances are often those who can least afford it.

Not being an expert in construction, I am unsure why my patients who live in mobile homes have so much trouble. It may be that fumes from construction adhesives and insulation are trapped in them. It may be that too much moisture penetrates the home through the floor.

I advise my patients to avoid living in mobile homes, if they can. If they must live in a home of this type, my only suggestion is to keep it as dry as possible by venting the area beneath the home to the outside and installing a moisture barrier over the cement or dirt on which it rests.

* * *

For those who suffer headaches, the age of their home and how it was constructed often determine how much pain they must endure. Try to keep these factors in mind as you search for a place to live.

What About All That Stuff in the Basement?

In the previous chapters, we talked about how soil moisture enters the home through the concrete slab, raises the humidity level in the area over the slab, and promotes the growth of excess house dust mites and mold—a major cause of the headaches that plague our patients.

Although soil moisture problems can be significantly reduced by proper site selection and landscape drainage, there is no way to prevent this moisture from penetrating the concrete slab that rests on the ground. Even "dry" soil contains a small amount of moisture. Proper site selection and landscape drainage are essential but do not guarantee moisture-free conditions.

Even if my patients could somehow install the perfect moisture barrier beneath their homes, who could say that this barrier wouldn't be compromised as the house ages and settles? Who could guarantee that the basement would never be flooded by a five-inch rainfall or a misdirected garden hose, or by any number of other natural or man-made catastrophes? No one could.

With these caveats in mind, the headache sufferer should follow two guiding principles in outfitting the basement:

- There is no way to guarantee a dry concrete slab.
- People with headaches must always assume the cement slab is wet and take appropriate action.

In light of these principles, what measures should the homeowner take? Let's try to answer this question.

Denying Shelter to Mites and Mold

Since a concrete floor in contact with the ground is never truly dry, homeowners must assume that the air above the slab is humid. They must therefore adopt any means to restrict the growth of dust mites and mold. They can do this by exploiting a weakness of these tiny organisms—their need for shelter. Knowing where they find this shelter and removing these items can often mean the difference between miserable headaches and a life free of head pain.

Carpeting

For dust mites and mold, carpeting lying on concrete is the promised land. In the pad beneath the carpet and in the carpet fibers, they find a warm dwelling place with a continuous supply of life-giving humidity.

Reducing the amount of carpeting in your home will diminish the amount of mold and dust mites that are harbored there. Avoid laying carpet on a concrete slab. If you must finish a basement floor, use tile or linoleum. If carpeting is your only option, avoid permanently installed carpeting that stretches wall to wall. Instead, use small area rugs, which are a far less inviting home for these pesky organisms. Not only can these rugs be removed for periodic cleaning, they are much easier and far less expensive to replace than wall-to-wall carpeting and padding.

Stuffed Furniture

Although you may relish the comfort of an overstuffed couch or recliner in your basement family room, remember that you are sharing such pleasures with a horde of unseen and unwanted guests. The materials used to stuff furniture soak up moisture like a sponge, and the coverings keep them from drying out.

If you must put chairs and sofas in an area with a concrete floor resting on the ground, use furniture with little or no padding. This will reduce the number of mites and mold growing in the area and will lessen their ability to stimulate head pain.

Storage

As we accrue years in a permanent residence, we also accumulate mountains of stored "treasure." Because the basement is a handy place to store our accumulated junk, it usually ends up there, neatly placed in cardboard boxes or other containers, ready for the day when we may need these little used items again.

Unfortunately, this treasure trove becomes another shelter for mites and mold. Often the items are so closely packed there is little room for air to circulate, so after they have become damp with humidity they are not likely to dry out. Since basement humidity levels are high enough to encourage microorganism growth throughout the year, and since cardboard boxes and their contents provide ample food for these tiny headache-causing microorganisms, they live contentedly. This happy situation for mites and mold is a disastrous one for their human housemates who are prone to headaches.

A good way to correct this situation is to pretend you are moving to a new home. Prepare for the move by sorting through all those treasures and getting rid of anything you would not take with you. Throw them out or give them away.

A week later, go back and do it again. After a month, do it again, and six months later, do it yet again. (If you're like me, you'll be surprised at how much there still is to get rid of.) Keep discarding until you have eliminated three-fourths of the material stored in your basement. Then, place what remains in plastic bags to keep the moisture out and any resident dust mites and mold in (metal, glass, wood, and plastic items need not be bagged in plastic).

Once you have reduced your stockpile of treasures to a small cluster of plastic bags, do not congratulate yourself just yet. Get yourself into the habit of repeating this process at least once every six months. Otherwise that demon pack rat inside you who just loves to store things in your basement will just clutter it up again.

Books

I love to read. I will read almost anything, from fiction to travel books, to medical journals—even the fine print on the toothpaste dispenser as I groggily brush my teeth in the morning. In the past, after reading a book I enjoyed, I would stow it away somewhere on the off chance a friend might ask for it or I myself would like to read it again in the future. At one time, I had walls of bookshelves filled with my favorite books, all lined up like soldiers standing at attention. But no more!

I discovered that, although the work of a good author ages well, the book in which it is printed doesn't. As it ages, it becomes damp and musty, providing a pleasant, food-laden home for mold. This is especially true for books stored in the basement. The constant elevated humidity there combines with the mild temperature to produce ideal conditions for the propagation of microorganisms that provoke headaches.

Don't allow your home to fill up with musty old books. First, throw out all the books you keep in the basement—they are no doubt moldy. Next, examine the books you keep in other parts of your home. Get rid of any you definitely won't ever read again. Then, reexamine the remaining books and throw out those you probably won't read again. After that, dispose of half of the remaining books, and finally, eliminate half of those you have left.

If you love reading as much as I do, this will hurt, but it is necessary if you want to feel better. However difficult it may be for you to give up your favorite books, believe me when I say you must do it. If you could only hear the stories of my many patients whose excruciating headaches persisted as long as they kept their prized collection of books, you would know how important it is for you to avoid the same mistake.

* * *

If you want to control your headaches or those of a loved one, focus your attention on your basement. My nurses and I do. We know that the basement is the greatest barrier to successfully treating our patients with headaches.

Stand in any area of your house where the floor is a concrete slab in contact with the ground. Look around for the problems we discussed and correct them, if possible.

When renting an apartment or purchasing a home, avoid those with living space above a concrete slab or garage. When the real estate agent shows you a house with a finished basement, you should smile, agree that the area is beautiful and the basement is dry, then leave this house and never return.

Dehumidifying the Basement

The rainy seasons of spring and fall increase groundwater levels, causing moisture to penetrate the basement floor and enter the house. This happens even in a house resting on sandy soil with perfect landscape drainage (if such a house exists). This moisture will turn into humidity that breeds mold and headaches.

Humidity also infiltrates the home from the outside air on humid days. With moisture from the air and slab, the basement acquires a peculiar odor. It smells musty.

This musty smell spells trouble. Although the homeowner often does not smell the mustiness in his basement or notice any dampness, it's there all the same. Mold grows in this air like it grows on a slice of damp bread. Once established, even the dryness of winter won't rid the basement of these microorganisms. Any activity in the living area above the slab launches mold into the air to be breathed by the headache sufferer.

At the same time that rainy, humid weather encourages mold growth, it also enables house dust mites to flourish. Even though mites dehydrate and die in winter's dryness, their bodies and fecal droppings remain behind, and any activity in the areas involved raises house dust contaminated by these substances. This dust also causes headaches. Thus, fighting the headaches of winter begins in spring, summer, and fall. Your best weapon for fighting them is a dehumidifier.

How a Dehumidifier Works

A dehumidifier is a device that blows warm moist air against coils of metal kept cool by a liquid circulating through them. It is actually a little refrigerator without the surrounding insulated box. The moisture in the air condenses on the coils and drips into a pan. This collected moisture is emptied periodically by the homeowner or allowed to run through a hose into a drain.

By drying the air, the dehumidifier robs mites and molds of the humidity necessary for unrestrained growth. It does not stop all growth, but it prevents the excessive numbers of mites and mold that stimulate pain in those who are prone to headaches.

Can the dehumidifier fail to keep mite and mold levels down? Yes, it is ineffective in the following situations:

- Some basements are so wet that a dehumidifier cannot adequately dry them. Correct the excess moisture problem by some other means, such as landscape drainage, or consider moving.

- The dehumidifier cannot dry a carpet and pad resting on a concrete floor that in turn rests upon the ground. It can only dry the air after it rises above them. The carpet and pad continue to be moist and continue to grow mites and mold. Consider removing wall-to-wall carpeting and replacing it with tile and throw rugs that can be removed for cleaning.

- It cannot dry stuffed furniture resting on a concrete floor. Moisture will penetrate the furniture before it evaporates into the basement air to be dried by the dehumidifier. Use furniture with little or no padding.

- Rooms in a basement separated by partitions are difficult to dehumidify. Avoid partitioning the basement into separate rooms.

- A dehumidifier cannot help if you do not use it.

Use the dehumidifier all through the year except when the cool midwinter temperatures and dry air would cause the machine to freeze up (cold, dry air causes ice to form on the coils). In the northern plains states, it should run continually from the end of March through November.

The dehumidifier is indispensable for my patients with headaches. One should be installed in every basement.

Part IV
The Rest of the House

The Upstairs Bedroom

When I first began treating allergic headaches, I was not aware of the importance of the home environment. It was only after years of experience that I realized excess moisture, house dust mites, and mold in the home must be reduced before I could treat my patients effectively.

Having grasped the need to modify conditions in the home, I then tried to determine what changes needed to be made. At first, it seemed obvious that I should concentrate my attention on the bedroom—after all, my patients spend hours there every night while they sleep. Because of the huge amount of time spent in this room, there is no doubt the bedroom air must have a profound effect on their headaches. I became an evangelist for the "allergy-proof" bedroom. "Allergy-proof your bedroom and you will conquer your headaches," I preached.

Surprisingly, the results were disappointing. Patient after patient told me allergy-proofing the bedroom did not help—they were just as uncomfortable as before.

What was wrong? Why did this seemingly sound advice fail? I came to realize that it failed because of the humidity rising from the concrete floor of the house. As long as the allergens bred by this humidity remained unchecked, allergy-proofing the bedroom provided little relief to the headache sufferer.

Trying to allergy-proof the bedroom while ignoring the basement is like trying to disinfect the bathroom by washing the window while ignoring the floor, bathtub, and toilet bowl. The bathroom would be far from clean. To fight our patients' headaches, we must first fight the humidity that rises from the concrete slab. That's why thus far we have concentrated on measures to correct allergen exposure in the basement.

However, just as the bathroom would not be completely clean unless you cleaned the window, it would be a mistake to ignore the bedroom in fighting the battle against headaches. If the growth of mold and mites is not fought vigorously throughout the house, headache control will be stymied. Patients will continue to suffer.

In an effort to avoid this mistake, let's look at what can be done to fight headaches caused by allergic exposures in the bedroom.

Correcting Problems in the Upstairs Bedroom

There seems to be no definitive reason why we humans need to sleep. It could be that, eons ago, the divine caretaker programmed those hulking ancestors of ours this way to keep them from roaming around at night and being devoured by some huge nocturnal carnivore. I suspect that since we still require regular slumber, this kindly caretaker continues to doubt our ability to stay out of trouble and thinks we are safer tucked in our beds at night.

Whatever the reason, the bedroom is the place where most of us satisfy this need, and we spend nearly a third of our lives there. The question is: What do we breathe in the air that surrounds us as we sleep?

The air in an upstairs bedroom contains the same unwanted guests we talked about when we discussed the basement bedroom—dust mites and mold. They choose the same hiding places—the mattress, pillow, bedclothing, stuffed furniture, and carpet—which provide them with comforting warmth and nourishing food.

All of us are forced to live with mites and mold. They are a fact of life whether we are sloppy housekeepers with "woolies" under the bed or compulsive cleaners with such immaculate homes that visitors are discouraged from entering without taking their shoes off at the door. However, although we must play host to these unwanted guests, we need not be gracious hosts.

The bedroom is one place where it is difficult to discourage mites and molds by denying them warmth—who wants to sleep in freezing temperatures? (Although, I have to admit, it is interesting how many of us who like to be warm when we sleep marry spouses who like the bedroom so cold it would make a polar bear shiver.) However, we can attack their need for shelter and moisture.

Denying Shelter and Moisture to Mites and Mold

Since preventing these tiny guests from sharing our bedrooms is impossible, isn't it fortunate that it is also unnecessary. Headaches strike only when their numbers are excessive—more than my patients can tolerate. Even the most severely affected headache sufferer can tolerate the small numbers found in a bedroom that is properly cared for. There are a number of factors that make this room either a refuge for mites and mold or a place where they cannot thrive. These factors include:

- The location of the bedroom;
- The type of bed coverings and their care;
- The condition of the mattress and pillow.

THE LOCATION OF THE BEDROOM. We have already discussed the inadvisability of locating bedrooms in the basement. For our patients with frequent headaches, sleeping in the basement is like a cow sleeping in a meat-packing plant: If the cow had any sense, it would sleep elsewhere. I cannot overemphasize how important it is for those who are plagued with headaches to sleep somewhere other than the basement.

The best bedroom location is on the first or second floor—the higher the better. Avoid any room where the floor is a concrete slab touching the ground. Also, avoid a bedroom that is situated over a crawl space or a garage.

THE TYPE OF BED COVERINGS AND THEIR CARE. It is best to replace feather, kapok, and cotton comforters with those made of synthetic fibers. Although mold and dust mites will grow in any material, including synthetic fibers, they grow better in natural materials. Bedding should be washed frequently and in hot water; cool-water washing does not kill mites.

THE CONDITION OF THE MATTRESS AND PILLOW. We spend a third of our lives in intimate contact with our mattress and pillow. If they are filled with mites and mold, they will cause headaches.

Is there a way to estimate their mite and mold content? Although there is no sure way to know whether a mattress or pillow harbors excess dust mites and mold, the following questions will help:

- *How old are they?* It is a fact of nature that we humans shed our skin in the form of dander or scales. This process continues when we are asleep, perspiring and tossing and turning in our beds. Therefore, years of use probably mean the bedding has acquired increased numbers of mites and mold. They live on discarded scales.

- *Where have they been stored or used?* It is important to think about where your bedding may have been stored or used in the past. I remember a fellow physician whose daughter's severe asthma disappeared when he replaced her mattress. It had been stored in a basement.

- *Were they exposed to a vaporizer or humidifier?* Many of us have used these devices at one time or another. Vaporizers and humidifiers turn our bedrooms into tropical rain forests, encouraging luxuriant microorganism growth in pillows and mattresses.

- *Have the mattress or pillows been used in an overinsulated house?* In an overinsulated, poorly ventilated house, there is too much moisture permeating the atmosphere everywhere, including the bedrooms.

If the answer to these questions indicates conditions favorable to mite and mold growth, either replace the mattress and pillow or encase them in airtight, zippered plastic covers. Such plastic coverings can be purchased at a store that sells bedding products or by contacting your local allergist for the names of companies that specialize in making mattress and pillow enclosures for the allergic patient.

Although replacement of a mattress can be financially draining, most of us can afford to buy new pillows every once in awhile. A good rule of thumb is to replace them every two years. Be sure to choose hypoallergenic pillows made of synthetic materials (dacron or foam). Eliminate feather pillows—mites and mold grow well in them.

Before leaving the subject of the bedroom, I should mention water beds. I suspect that they may worsen my patients' symptoms. Sometimes a problem is obvious—a small leak that causes a green or black stain on the bedcovers or mattress. At other times, there is no obvious leak, but my patient's headaches are unusually painful and frequent and I can find no other environmental reason for this degree of suffering. Although I am concerned that the water bed is causing these symptoms, I have no proof that it does so.

* * *

Proper care of the bedroom reduces the levels of house dust mites and mold that live there and reduces the headaches of those who sleep there. Any changes made here, added to other changes in your home, should reward you with pleasing headache relief.

Carpets, Bathrooms, Plants, Aquariums, Hot Tubs, etc.

As my nurses and I take our mental inventory of the typical house, searching for high concentrations of house dust mites and mold, we look for places and things that provide the moisture and shelter conditions that encourage their growth. Our years of experience have led us to attach more significance to certain conditions and to be more forceful in encouraging our patients to change them.

Many of the suggestions for change that follow are generally accepted by other allergists, but there is disagreement about some of these recommendations among my colleagues. Whether a particular piece of advice is generally accepted or somewhat controversial, we find it works.

Carpets

You will recall from our discussion of how mites and mold find moisture and shelter in basement carpet that I strongly recommended removing it and replacing it with tile or area rugs. But what about carpeting in the rest of the house? Wouldn't it seem logical to remove this carpeting, too?

Although it seems logical, it probably isn't necessary. My patients do not appear to be bothered by carpets installed on the first and second floors of a house except in certain instances. In determining whether these carpets need to be removed, the following should be considered:

- How old is it?
- What is under it?
- Can it be cleaned?

HOW OLD IS IT? New carpets release fumes that many of my patients find disagreeable. These fumes usually disappear in six to twelve months, but while they are present, they can cause headaches. Lay new carpeting in the spring so it can air out through the summer. If a home is poorly ventilated, laying new carpet in the winter can lead to irritating symptoms.

The older the carpeting, the more likely it is to cause headaches. Many patients have told me their headaches improved immensely when old carpeting was replaced. I suspect that as carpeting gets older, its fibers begin to flake and are released into the air as an irritating dust. How can you tell whether carpeting is old? I'm not sure, but if it looks old and your headaches are bothersome, get rid of it.

If you move into a home where a dog or cat has lived, the carpet may have become contaminated by animal dander, saliva, urine, and feces. You should seriously consider removing this carpeting.

WHAT IS UNDER IT? Carpets resting on a floor that has no contact with the ground should be dry and relatively free of mites and mold. They should not be a major cause of headaches, and I do not believe they need to be replaced. For this reason, I do not discourage carpeting in upstairs rooms that are dry.

This is not the case in the poorly ventilated home. Here, the moisture from breathing, cooking, bathing, dishwashing, laundering, and other activities builds to high levels throughout the house, and the carpeting on all floors is bathed in the humidity we strive so hard to defeat in the basement. This house must be ventilated or the carpeting should be removed.

The same growth occurs in any area of the house with high humidity. Carpeting in bathrooms and any area subject to humidification is unwise. Carpeting should be removed from a room where a humidifier or vaporizer was used if the homeowner suspects it causes headaches.

CAN IT BE CLEANED? This question applies only to carpeting in humid areas of the house, such as the basement. There, floor coverings should be limited to tile or small area rugs that can be removed easily for cleaning.

The value of cleaning was researched by McDonald and Tovey, who reported their findings in the *Journal of Allergy and Clinical Immunology* in October of 1992. They found that cold-water washing reduced the mite allergen (the part of the mite that causes allergy) concentration by more than ninety percent, but live mites were not destroyed. Dry cleaning killed the mites but did not remove enough of their bodies or droppings. All mites were killed and significantly removed by washing in water at a temperature of 55 degrees Celsius or higher (131 degrees Fahrenheit). The hot-water wash is the cleaning method most effective in killing and removing mites.

Wall-to-wall carpeting is less desirable than small area rugs because it is permanently installed and cannot be removed to be beaten or cleaned. In an attempt to reduce its content of mite allergen (the part of the mite that causes allergy), tannic acid and benzyl benzoate products have been developed. The American College of Allergy and Immunology, in a leaflet entitled "House Dust Allergies Common Even in Clean Homes," describes these products:

Tannic acid can be sprayed on carpets or upholstered furniture to break down allergen from mites and cat dander. When the allergen is inactivated, it can no longer cause allergy symptoms. Tannic acid works fast and is easy to use, but its effects do not last long because mites remain and allergen continues to build up, requiring frequent application of the product. Also, some people have complained it may stain some carpets and upholstery fabrics.

To kill mites, benzyl benzoate moist powder can be brushed into carpets, allowed to dry for 8 to 12 hours, and vacuumed up. The Environmental Protection Agency (EPA) has approved this product as safe for home use, and it will not usually stain carpets. Unlike tannic acid, benzyl benzoate's effect is long-lasting. After one or two initial applications, you can keep mites and your symptoms under control by using it only once or twice a year.

I find I am uncomfortable with the use of these products. Tannic acid is only effective for a short time and does not kill the house dust mite—it continues to grow. Even though the EPA finds benzyl benzoate safe for home use, I am concerned about the long-term health effects of exposure to a product that kills mites.

Is use of these products necessary if the carpet is in good shape and used in a dry room? I do not believe so. By using these products, can the homeowner avoid removing carpeting from moist areas of the house? No; I believe that such carpeting should be removed.

The marketers of tannic acid and benzyl benzoate do not advertise their products as mold inhibitors. Even though they kill mites, if they do not kill these other organisms, their continued growth will still cause the headaches we are trying to stop.

I can think of two instances where benzyl benzoate may be useful. The headache sufferer may be forced to rent a basement apartment or other living quarters with carpeting that has been affected by moisture. If the carpet cannot be replaced, it should be treated to kill mites. Also, in cases where the homeowner cannot immediately remove a carpet from an area that is moist, the carpet can be treated until it can be removed.

For information on where to purchase tannic acid and benzyl benzoate carpet products, contact your primary doctor or allergist.

Bathrooms

Showering and bathing produce much of the humidity the headache sufferer must contend with. This humidity should be eliminated in some way, especially in the super-insulated home. A moisture-activated fan vented to the outside should accomplish this task well.

The bathroom often conceals a major problem for the headache sufferer. Over years of use, a defect can develop in the walls or floor, allowing moisture to penetrate them and causing areas of rot. This rot can be hidden and almost impossible to find; we can only suspect it when unusually frequent and severe headaches persist in spite of our treatment.

On a number of occasions, my patients have gained precious relief from their head pain after replacing floors and walls that have rotted. As with rot caused by roof and vent leaks, the homeowner should be constantly on the alert for areas that may have rotted due to bathroom moisture.

The basement shower is of great concern to me. A ten-minute stay in a musty shower can cause severe headaches that may not appear until hours later and may last for days. People with headaches should not use a basement shower. They should not even live in a home that has one. Although the highest levels of mold will be found in the shower, its mustiness will permeate the entire house.

Plants

I once dreamed of owning a home with an attached greenhouse where I could spend my leisure hours growing flowers and vegetables. Short of that, I wanted a home filled with plants. Unfortunately, because of my allergies, I have had to forego these dreams.

Every plant is a miniature moisture factory, constantly humidifying the air and contributing to the growth of dust mites and mold. The soil that nourishes the plant also nourishes mold. Because plants make our homes so attractive and give us so much pleasure, they tend to be overlooked as enemies in the fight to keep humidity down.

A patient whose house contains a large number of plants will find headaches difficult to treat. However, not all plants need be eliminated. Limit the number to five average-sized plants for a home, less for an apartment. Never place any plants in the bedroom. Your head will be better off.

Aquariums

As I once dreamed of tending plants in my greenhouse, I also dreamed of tending tropical fish in an aquarium. Someday, I hoped, the mystery and beauty of the brightly colored fish in the pet stores I frequented would be mine to enjoy at home. Unfortunately, my allergies also put an end to this dream.

As with plants, the aquarium is a moisture factory. If it has an aerator, the air escaping from the tank also carries with it the algae and other microorganisms growing in the aquarium, and this air causes trouble.

I discovered this when treating a boy for nasal congestion and headaches whose symptoms were frustratingly persistent. Only when the ten-gallon aquarium was removed from his bedroom did his nose return to normal. Many other patients have suffered similar congestion and headaches that also improved when an aquarium was removed.

I believe that a small goldfish bowl without an aerator, situated in a living room or other large area of the home, is probably acceptable in most cases, but a large aquarium with an aerator is never acceptable. If the headache sufferer wants relief, the aquarium must go.

Hot Tubs

Two other sources of the humidity that encourages mite and mold growth are hot tubs and pools situated inside a house or apartment. I realize they are popular ways of relaxing in today's stressful lifestyle, but in my opinion these reservoirs of standing warm water should have warning signs that read: "Danger: May cause headaches." Just as with vaporizers and humidifiers, we should strive to eliminate these moisture sources. I find it discouraging to start a regimen of headache treatment when a patient lives in a building with one of these humidity producers. All of our dietary, environmental, and injection treatments may fail in these cases. My best advice is:

- Don't buy a house or rent an apartment with a hot tub or pool.
- If you own a home with one, drain it and dry it out.
- Disconnect the plumbing so it cannot be used.
- Use it to store objects that aren't susceptible to mold.

Humidifiers

Years ago, when I first entered practice, I found myself treating large numbers of asthmatics who were very sick. For these unfortunate people, just staying out of the hospital was a major accomplishment, and one they found difficult to achieve. I was fresh out of allergy training, and although my head was filled with the *scientific* knowledge my instructors had worked so diligently to teach me, I hadn't yet acquired the *practical* knowledge that comes from working with patients in a clinical setting. I wrestled with the problem of trying to figure out why their illness was so devastating for a long time, until it finally dawned on me that they all had one thing in common. They lived, ate, and slept in a fog of water from using vaporizers or humidifiers.

You might be asking yourself: What's so wrong with that? I asked myself this same question, since it was common practice at the time for asthmatics to use such devices to alleviate breathing problems. But when I checked the scientific literature, I learned that many of the germs that cause pneumonia live in humidifier and vaporizer water and are dispersed into the fog they create.

I was so intrigued by this information that I decided to do some experimenting. I took samples of water from vaporizers and humidifiers and cultured them to see whether they would grow mold. The water was loaded with mold spores! I even found the microorganisms that cause a type of lung-destroying pneumonia called farmer's lung.

Add to these pernicious germs the mites and mold that grow in the carpets, bedding, furniture, and clothes that are exposed to this high humidity and there is ample reason for the severe cases of asthma in my patients. When I strictly forbade the use of vaporizers and humidifiers, their dreadful asthma attacks subsided. This was definitely a case of the "cure" making the condition worse.

As the focus of my practice shifted more and more to the treatment of headaches, I found I needed to discourage the use of humidifiers and vaporizers for my patients to overcome their severe head pain. It is simply unwise for my patients to use them. I know that without humidity, the wood in furniture, pianos, and other valuable objects can dry out, warp, and split, but my patients must decide what is more important to them—preserving their furniture or improving their quality of life.

When the winters are especially dry, some of my patients will add moisture to their homes by boiling water on the stove. If this is not overdone, I do not object. Others will run a vaporizer for a half hour to help a coughing child go to sleep. If the vaporizer is then washed out with soap and hot water and put away, again I do not object. If the child being treated with the vaporizer is an allergic child, prolonged exposure to vaporized water—and to the mite and mold growing in a humidified room—may only lead to increased illness.

Patients often tell me their houses are so dry that their noses and throats become dry and irritated—they need to use a humidifier to counteract this dryness. I believe they are missing the point. If they lived in a desert with humidity lower than that found in their homes, their throats and noses would be fine. It is not the dryness that is causing these miserable symptoms. The mites and mold growing in their homes irritate their noses and throats, and it is this irritation that makes them feel dry. To relieve these symptoms, don't turn on the humidifier or vaporizer. Correct the environment instead.

Vaporizers and humidifiers quickly become loaded with a bewildering variety of germs, and these organisms make the water in them extremely unhealthy. You would never drink this water, so why would you vaporize it and then breathe it? Which translates to a principle I strongly believe in: *Never vaporize water you would not drink.* This principle translates into the following warning: *If you have headaches, never use a vaporize or humidifier.*

Firewood

The logs we burn in our fireplaces are old and moldy. In addition, many of the molds are types that allergists do not test for or treat. Therefore, it is not a good idea to dry or store them in the home.

Wood smoke is a dangerous pollutant and does not belong in the home. From my observations of patients who have wood furnaces, no matter how efficient they are, some smoke always seems to end up in the house. I do not believe patients with headaches should heat their homes with wood.

Woodburning fireplaces also produce pollutants. They should be drafted well, with combustion air entering from the outside and an efficient glass door over the opening to reduce the amount of smoke and odor that enters the living area. Any enjoyment and relaxation they may afford the occupants of the home will be quickly overshadowed if they bring on pain for those who are prone to headaches.

Clothes Dryers

A major thrust of this book is to lower the moisture in the headache sufferer's environment. Air drying wet clothes in the basement cancels many of the actions the homeowner takes to dry the house. Use a clothes dryer, but do not vent the dryer into the basement. Vent it to the outside. I've cultured the air from clothes dryers and found that it is loaded with yeast. Breathing air loaded with yeast can only mean trouble for the headache sufferer.

* * *

In this chapter, we looked at many conditions that frustrate our treatment of headaches. If any of these conditions are present in your home, and you want to relieve your headaches, I strongly recommend that you change them. It really helps.

Part V
Other
Exposures

Pets and Pollens

In the previous chapters, we concentrated our efforts on learning how moisture in the home produces excessive levels of house dust mites that cause sinus, migraine, and cluster headaches. But our knowledge of headache causes will not be complete if we focus only on these potent sources of headaches and ignore other major sources. Two of these other sources are the pets owned by so many of us and the pollens we all breathe in summer. Pollens are major instigators of headache, but pets probably are not.

Pets

For those who own and love a Tabby or a Spot, I have pleasant news. Although I believe that dog and cat exposures cause allergic headaches, I do not believe they are the most important causes.

This does not mean that exposure to pets does not precipitate allergy symptoms, because it does. Nor does it mean pet exposure cannot trigger headaches, because it can. The presence of a pet is always regrettable in the home of the allergic person. In giving rise to wheezing, stuffy noses, itchy skin and hives, and other allergic illnesses, cats and dogs belong in the major leagues, but—as far as I can determine—in their ability to provoke headaches, they are only in the minor leagues.

Why do I think so? One reason is that we treat many patients who live with dogs and cats, and our treatment stops their headaches, even though their nasal stuffiness or wheezing persists. Often these latter symptoms will continue until that day when the pet is no longer in the picture. So headaches are treatable, despite the presence of a pet in the home.

Another reason is the experiences of my patients whose pets have died. When I ask them if their headaches improved after their pet's death, although the answer is sometimes yes, most often the answer is no.

I confess I may be biased in this regard. When I first began practicing allergy, I refused to treat patients unless they got rid of their pets. To this day, I remember the tears of the children when I issued this prudent—but heartless—dictate. My resolve melted at their sad little faces and reproachful eyes. I decided to allow patients to keep their pets, and to my surprise, most of the time, the treatment works well.

Still another reason is that I believe pet allergy does not worsen with time. Although this belief is not as well founded as I might wish, I still hold it firmly. If a patient has headaches today, even though he or she continues to live with a dog or cat, there will be no increase in the frequency or severity of their head pain a year from now.

This is in sharp contrast to the progressive increase in headaches when high levels of moisture, mold, and house dust mites are involved. Headaches strike more frequently and more painfully and must be fought more vigilantly. The home must be kept as dry as possible.

Please do not use what I have just said to justify adding a cat or dog to your household. As you can probably guess, I am still struggling with my decision to treat patients who refuse to give up their animals. It may be that my desire to spare my patients the heart-rending sorrow of parting with their beloved pets has blinded me to the truth about their potential to cause headaches. Please do not compound the difficulty of treating your headaches by bringing a dog or cat into your home.

Minimizing the Impact of Having a Pet

Even though a pet packs less headache potential than mold and dust mites, it is wise to minimize this potential. If the pet does not live in the house, exposure is minimal. Keeping a dog outside is the ideal solution. However, if a pet is kept inside the house, certain actions can be taken to reduce exposure to the saliva, urine, dander, and hair that carry dog and cat allergens.

Some of these measures are obvious: avoid holding and petting the animal; do not allow it into the bedroom; restrict it to only one part of the house. But there are other helpful steps that can be taken.

A number of studies have looked at ways to reduce cat allergen, and their findings may also hold true for dog allergen. They show that bathing a cat weekly dramatically reduces the amount of allergen it sheds. They also show that carpeted rooms hold far more cat allergen than rooms with bare floors. In fact, air cleaners only reduce the level of cat allergen in rooms without carpeting. Room furnishings such as drapes or curtains, stuffed furniture, and other dust collectors also increase the level of cat allergen. The following steps can be effective in reducing cat allergen:

- Washing the cat weekly;
- Removing furnishings, drapes, or curtains;
- Removing carpeting;
- Using an air cleaner.

For the allergic family determined to keep a pet, these suggestions will reduce exposure to its allergens and thus reduce the discomfort it causes.

One last suggestion—it is probably wise to get into the habit of washing your hands after touching your pet. Animal saliva contains much of the allergen that bothers sensitive people. Cats become covered with this saliva as they groom themselves. Dogs are not only showing their affection by licking their masters' hands and faces, they are also leaving behind allergens.

Pollens

I can't imagine anyone appreciating springtime more than those of us who live in the northern states. At last, we can throw open the windows and let its cleansing breezes air out our stuffy houses and warm our spirits.

But we shouldn't let these enchanting breezes fool us into believing we have left our headaches behind. They often bring head pain that is equally as severe as that we endure in winter.

Tiny passengers called pollens ride the breezes of spring, summer, and fall, searching for plants just like their parents. Each bit of pollen is the male sperm of a tree, a grass, or a weed, and its mission is to mate with a female egg from a plant of the same species. Together they form a fertilized egg that grows into a new plant.

Each plant releases its pollen at a particular time of year, depending on the area of the country in which it grows. In the southern states, with their prolonged warm weather, the pollen season is also prolonged, with plants slowly releasing pollen throughout most of the year. This is not so in the northern states, where pollen must be released quickly because the growing season is so short.

In these northern states, trees shed billions of tiny pollens into the winds during April and May. June's sunny warmth prompts grasses to pollinate, while July stimulates the release of pollen from many weeds. The winds of August and September carry ragweed pollen—as so many hay fever sufferers can bitterly attest—until the first frost puts an end to their flight.

As we learned in our grade-school science classes, wind-borne pollination is nature's way of reproducing the green plants so necessary to our lives. We could not survive without the process of photosynthesis, which produces the oxygen we need for breathing. However, breathing pollens prompts headaches in many people who are sensitive to them. As we learned in our discussion of how allergy causes headaches, the immune system mistakenly thinks the harmless pollens are deadly germs. In the ensuing battle, the immune system triggers pain somewhere in the head.

Years ago, because the sneezing, wheezing, and eye swelling caused by pollens occurred at the same time hay was growing and being harvested, these symptoms came to be known as hay fever. We still use this term today.

There Is No Mystery

There should be no mystery in determining the cause of headaches when they strike year after year during the spring, summer, and fall pollen seasons. But it's frustrating how many people do not recognize this pattern. Time and again, I interview patients who have suffered years of summer headaches. No one—neither primary doctor nor patient—noticed the obvious cause.

Why was it missed? It certainly wasn't due to ignorance about when pollen levels are at their highest, because local television and radio weather programs and newspapers report the pollen count each day during the pollen seasons. It would be understandable if these headaches were rare, but they are not. Most of my patients with hay fever experience headaches during the pollen seasons, and since hay fever affects many people, such headaches are common.

The most likely reason for missing the role pollen plays in causing headaches is also a simple one. Doctors tend to search—as they should—for tumors, aneurysms, high blood pressure, or other causes of head pain that threaten a patient's health or life. When they find no evidence of any major disorder, they are relieved and search no further. Patients also feel relieved just to have the doctor name the type of headache they are experiencing: "migraine," or "sinus," or "tension." They, too, search no further.

But the search should not end there. Naming the type of headache does not tell *why* it arises, only *where* it arises—migraine headaches from the blood vessels of the head, cluster headaches from the nerves of the face and scalp, sinus headaches from the sinus cavities, and tension headaches from the muscles of the neck or forehead. When these migraine, sinus, cluster, or tension headaches appear during the tree, grass, or ragweed pollen seasons, both doctor and patient should question whether they are caused or aggravated by these pollens. Only when pollens are recognized as the cause of these headaches can effective allergy treatment be received.

Treating Summer Headaches

Whether headaches are mild or severe, simple measures can often provide relief, and we will touch briefly on them here. Severe headaches may require allergy injections in addition to medications, and we will discuss these injections in a later chapter.

AVOIDING POLLEN. No method of treating allergy is more effective than avoidance. If pollen is avoided, pollen headaches are avoided. Air conditioning, air cleaning, closing the bedroom window at night, and staying out of fields where plants are pollinating work well. Staying cooped up in the house all summer is an effective measure, but so draconian that anyone who is forced to do so should consider allergy injections.

NONPRESCRIPTION ANTIHISTAMINES AND DECONGESTANTS. These are convenient and your first line of drug treatment. They can often provide relief without the annoyance of having to obtain a doctor's prescription. Try several different types to find one that helps you. These medications are usually effective for mild to moderate hay fever; they may fail to relieve more severe symptoms. Ask your physician or pharmacist for suggestions. Be sure to read all the directions and cautions on the package, and do not use these medicines if you have a medical condition such as high blood pressure that may be worsened by taking them. Many people experience drowsiness from using these drugs, making work and driving dangerous. If they cause sleepiness or other distressing reactions, don't take them.

PRESCRIPTION ANTIHISTAMINES AND DECONGESTANTS. The newer antihistamines can only be obtained by prescription at this time—consult your physician. Although often more expensive than nonprescription drugs, they may cause less drowsiness, and they usually work well.

CORTISONE NASAL SPRAYS. These prescription sprays help many with severe hay fever, but for others they provide little relief. They do not seem to damage the nose or cause ill effects elsewhere in the body if used as directed. Use these sprays strictly according to your doctor's instructions, and report any adverse effects immediately.

CROMOLYN NASAL SPRAYS. Often used instead of cortisone nasal sprays, cromolyn sprays must be used consistently and on a continuous basis for them to work. It seems wise to begin using this prescription medication two weeks before the pollen season starts and to continue it daily throughout the season.

NONPRESCRIPTION NASAL SPRAYS. These can be helpful if used infrequently for severe nasal congestion. However, it is easy to overuse them, and your nose can become extremely stuffy, a condition called rebound. It is difficult to pinpoint when overuse occurs, but it is likely to happen if you use them for more than three days in a row or if you reuse them without giving your nose sufficient time to recover from the last use. Be sure to follow label cautions and directions.

CORTISONE TABLETS. Cortisone is a prescription medicine used by doctors to abort a severe attack of hay fever brought on by huge amounts of pollen at the peak of the season. It is also used when a cold (viral upper respiratory infection) makes hay fever symptoms go wild. This potent medication must be used only as prescribed.

This is only an overview of the medications that are available to help relieve hay fever and hopefully blunt the headaches that can accompany it. Providing a detailed description would make this book impossibly long. Directions on the use of nonprescription medicine should come from the information supplied with the medication or from your pharmacist. Guidance on the use of prescription medications must come only from your physician.

* * *

Although we spent a great deal of time examining the role of moisture, mold, and house dust mites in causing headaches and only part of a chapter discussing the role of pollens, this doesn't mean that pollens are not a significant factor. They cause distressing headaches for millions of people. It simply means that moisture, mold, and mites are far less obvious factors, and much more explanation is required to convince patients they might be the cause of their headaches and to describe the complicated measures necessary to defeat them.

Pollens are easier to suspect, and many common remedies are available to reduce their impact. Think of them if you or a loved one has recurring spring, summer, or fall headaches.

Smoking

Smoking rates a chapter by itself, not because the effects of smoke are complicated to describe, but because they are grave. However, the message is so simple that the chapter requires only one page. My patients tell me that smoking causes headaches. If you have headaches frequently, you should not smoke.

Smokers should not smoke around people who are susceptible to headaches. Passive smoke will permeate every room in a building where smoking is allowed. My advice to smokers is unequivocal:

- Do not smoke in the basement.
- Do not smoke on the first floor.
- Do not smoke on the second floor.
- Do not smoke in the office.
- Do not smoke at meetings.
- Do not smoke at parties.
- Do not smoke in the car (even if the windows are open).
- Do not smoke in any area where your smoke will affect those who suffer from headaches.
- If you must smoke, do it outdoors.

Headaches at Work

The mold and house dust mites that live in the home concern me, and I believe my concern is warranted. Years of treating patients with miserable headaches convinces me these moisture-loving microorganisms are major causes of the pain my patients suffer. I can almost visualize the house dust mites and mold growing abundantly in the homes of these patients, as vigorously as plants grow in a greenhouse, and for the same reasons—warm air, humidity, shelter, and food.

But not all headaches arise from the home. Many patients suffer from headaches caused by the buildings in which they work. In fact, work-related headaches and other symptoms occur so frequently that they have been given a special name—the "sick building syndrome."

I am not an expert on the sick building itself. Those with knowledge of building design, construction, ventilation, and all the other features of a building must be looked to as the experts. However, because I treat patients who work in sick buildings, I am an expert in the illnesses they

147

cause. These illnesses affect many of my patients, making it appropriate to discuss them here.

A good way to examine the sick building syndrome is to review an article from the June 29, 1992, edition of the Saint Paul *Pioneer Press* by Scott Carlson entitled, "Does Your Work Make You Sick?" Let's look at the information he gathered.

The Number of People Affected

A random survey of two hundred Minneapolis workers by Harris Research found that more than seven in ten respondents said they experienced health problems associated with their workplace. Furthermore, an official with the Minnesota Department of Health quoted a World Health Organization estimate that thirty percent of new and remodeled buildings have problems related to the sick building syndrome.

Do you think these figures are exaggerated? I don't. Many of my patients tell me they suffer from painful headaches on the job, making going to work a dreaded ordeal. To my mind, this is another example of our ingenuity outpacing our good sense. Like the small child who learns to strike a match but does not know how to put out a fire, we have developed high-technology computer systems to control the mechanical aspects of the ventilation systems in commercial buildings, but we often fail to deliver air that is healthy for the employees who work in them to breathe.

When we "tighten up" our workplaces to reduce the cost of heating and cooling, we substitute "technologically" conditioned air for the healthful ventilation nature provides. If we make mistakes, our employees become ill. As we reduce heating and cooling costs, we increase the costs of medical care and employee absenteeism due to illness.

The sick building syndrome has an enormous impact on my patients. Too many of them work in buildings that cause miserable headaches.

What Makes Buildings Sick?

For this information, we can turn to the experience of Healthy Buildings International (HBI), which reviewed 813 buildings with 750,000 occupants. They studied the major causes of problems, the pollutants and problems found, and the effect on employees. The lists on the following page describe their findings.

HBI surveyed two hundred Minneapolis workers at random, asking them whether they had health problems associated with the sick building syndrome. Their survey agreed with that of Harris Research—more than seven out of ten answered affirmatively. That is a lot of people.

What Does It All Mean?

The information in the table teaches several valuable lessons. First, only experts in building construction and maintenance can reliably inspect and evaluate a building for symptoms of sick building syndrome. The bad air in a building can be attributed to a number of things, including faulty design or construction, faulty operations and maintenance, and less than optimum use of the ventilating system. Because the health of the occupants is at stake, it is imperative that the inspection be performed competently. The inspectors' credentials should be thoroughly checked before they check out the building.

The second lesson is that all kinds of pollutants and problems can be found in a sick building, and the most common are those familiar to allergists—dust, moisture, molds, and polluted air. Allergists are also familiar with the symptoms affecting the occupants of sick buildings, because these are the symptoms our patients bring to us for treatment.

Headaches, tiredness, listlessness, irritability, dry, watery, or itchy eyes, stuffy or runny noses, dry or sore throats, and flu-like illnesses—these are among the symptoms reported by people who work in sick buildings. These same symptoms can be caused by any of the buildings our patients occupy, which are also susceptible to faulty construction and operation, including the homes they live in.

Major Causes of Problems	(Percent of Buildings)
Operating faults and/or poor maintenance	75.6
Inefficient filtration of air supply	56.9
Poor ventilation due to energy conservation	54.1
Poor air distribution	20.8
Design errors	16.5
Contamination inside duct work	12.1

Pollutants and Problems Found	(Percent of Buildings)
Allergenic fungi	33.4
Dusts	26.6
Low relative humidity	18.5
Allergenic or pathogenic bacteria	10.2
Formaldehyde	8.5
Fibrous glass	6.6
Vehicle exhaust fumes	5.6
Volatile organic compounds	4.1
Tobacco smoke	2.8
High relative humidity	2.1
Ozone	1.0

Effect on Employees	(Percent of Survey Respondents with Symptoms)
Tiredness	54
Headache	40
Dry eyes	39
Dry throat	30
Watery or itchy eyes	19
Flu symptoms	19
Listlessness	16
Itchy or runny nose	15
No complaints	23

Understanding that both the home and work environments give rise to the same symptoms suggests a way to treat the patient plagued by sick building syndrome. This is illustrated by Sarah's story, which, although it does not involve a workplace, is a good example of all the sick buildings our patients encounter.

Sarah's Story

I met Sarah and her mother, Allison, as I was struggling with this chapter (struggling is a good description of the way I write). Sarah attends a high school far from home, and Allison brought her to see me during her summer vacation.

As Sarah sat in my office, it was easy to see that she was in need of help. Her eyes were swollen and her nose was obviously stuffy—she was constantly sniffing and breathing through her mouth. She looked miserable.

I felt sorry for this uncomfortable young woman. "Sarah, what brings you to see me?" I asked (as if it weren't painfully apparent).

"I feel crummy, Dr. Walsh," Sarah replied, sniffling once again. "I haven't felt good for the past year."

"What's been happening?" I asked, prompting her to tell me more, which she did in a flood of words.

"My nose is stuffed up. I constantly have this thick mucus in my throat that makes me sick. My throat and eyes feel dry and hurt a lot. I get headaches that start in the back of my neck and spread up over my scalp to my forehead and sometimes reach downward to my shoulders. And it seems like I have a cold all the time."

"And she is always tired and irritable," added Allison.

The symptoms listed by Sarah and Allison are classic examples of those that afflict people who work in a sick building. But Sarah's sick building is not her workplace, it's her dorm at school. Prior to moving to the dorm, she experienced only mild symptoms of allergy. Since she moved there, her discomfort has increased dramatically. Her distress was somewhat puzzling because she lives on the second floor—which should put her out of reach of the dust mites and mold on the lower floors. However, the building is old, and I suspect even the second floor is moist and populated with more mites and mold than she can tolerate.

To further add to Sarah's misery, when at home, she sleeps in the basement. Because of the high levels of moisture, mites, and mold there, for Sarah the house is a sick building. Even when she's on vacation from school, her miserable symptoms persist.

And if that isn't enough, Sarah's spends the summer weekends at her family's lake cabin, where she again encounters moisture, mites, and mold, causing further distress. Since she had recently returned from the cabin when she came to my office, it was no wonder she looked and felt so miserable.

Sarah's story is repeated countless times by other patients, many of whom find the workplace makes them ill. Is the sick building syndrome for real? Absolutely. Can a building make my patients sick? Yes, without doubt. Does the sick building exist only in the work environment? No. School, home, and the lake cabin can be equally to blame.

Perhaps the greatest lesson of Sarah's story is that patients with headaches must be aware of all the sick buildings in which they live, work, study, or vacation. If they are not, they will fail to recognize their combined impact on their headaches. They will also be unlikely to correct or avoid these conditions.

Recognizing the Sick Building Syndrome

There are four clues that help identify the sick building syndrome: the symptoms themselves; where and when they occur; and similar illnesses in other occupants of the building.

THE SYMPTOMS THEMSELVES. Look back at the symptoms found by HBI in its survey of people affected by the buildings in which they worked: headaches; recurrent colds or flu-like illnesses; dry or irritated and often painful throats, noses, and eyes. Together with tiredness and listlessness, these constitute a debilitating array of symptoms for these employees to cope with each day.

Although these symptoms sound too general to help diagnose the sick building syndrome, they are really very specific and readily identify it. We hear about this combination of symptoms so frequently that it has become familiar. When our patients describe them, we suspect that somewhere in their daily lives, they spend significant time in a building where they are exposed to high levels of allergens and pollutants. Because we hear so many of these stories, these multiple symptoms are not mysterious but have come to be expected in patients reacting to a sick building.

WHERE AND WHEN THEY OCCUR. The diagnosis of a sick building at work is helped immeasurably if symptoms start on one of the first days of the work week, Monday or Tuesday, and improve over the weekends or during vacation. If symptoms occur during the school year and improve during school vacation, the school may be implicated. If the home is at fault, the symptoms are more likely to occur daily and may not improve during vacation. After all, a two-week vacation may not reverse the harm caused by months or years of living in a sick home.

SIMILAR ILLNESSES IN OTHER BUILDING OCCUPANTS. If our patient is the only employee affected, he or she may be working in a sick building, but the lack of corresponding symptoms in other occupants makes the diagnosis shaky. Whenever the sick building syndrome is suspected, a search for similarly affected coworkers must be conducted to support the diagnosis.

In diagnosing the home as a sick building, it helps if other family members are similarly affected. However, this supporting evidence is often lacking because the number of people living in a home is small compared to the hundreds that may work in an office or factory. The more people occupying a building, the greater the chance that others will share the distressing symptoms that lead to a diagnosis of sick building syndrome.

Treating the Work-Related Headache

So far, I have spent a great deal of time describing the steps necessary to correct conditions at home that cause illnesses, especially headaches. But what can be done about conditions at work that cause similar illnesses?

Unfortunately, although we can recognize that our patients' illness are brought on by conditions at work, we often cannot do much to change the workplace. There are several reasons for this.

THE BUILDING'S FAULTS ARE OFTEN MISDIAGNOSED. Identifying why a building causes sickness seems like such a simple task—just call in the experts. However, many of my patients work for employers who *have* called in the experts *and* followed their advice to correct any problems. In spite of their good intentions, the work site still provokes miserable symptoms. This frustrating situation occurs all too often.

THE EMPLOYER MAY NOT BE ABLE TO FIX THE BUILDING. Many people work for marginally profitable businesses located in outdated buildings. The cost of modernizing the building may exceed the value of the business.

THE EMPLOYER MAY NOT WANT TO FIX THE BUILDING. Employees who find themselves in these circumstances have little choice. If they want to keep their jobs, they must be willing to live with their symptoms.

THE EMPLOYER MAY NOT BELIEVE THE BUILDING IS SICK. If this is the case, complaining employees may find themselves forced out of work or fired. Many of my patients know they cannot complain to the boss and continue to receive a paycheck.

Illness caused by a sick building is difficult to prove. The presence of broken bones can be proven with x-rays, and a diagnosis of lung damage can be corroborated with breathing tests. But there is no way to substantiate claims of headaches and tiredness. This lack of proof makes it hard to convince those with the authority to correct conditions in the sick building that the illness is real. It also makes it difficult, if not impossible, to collect worker's compensation benefits.

Employees should be very careful about informing the boss that the work site is making them ill. They should only do so if they are sure the employer will be sympathetic to their complaints. Before deciding to complain, it is always wise for a worker to search out others who are similarly affected and form a group to bring the problem to the attention of the employer. This will lessen the chance of any one member getting the reputation of being a chronic complainer. It is also unlikely that an entire group of employees would be fired.

What Can Be Done?

I wonder how many more studies will have to be done before employers begin to accept the reality of sick building syndrome. Until they do, my patients may be forced to accept illness to continue receiving their paychecks.

Although the situation often seems bleak and the prospect for treatment hopeless, this is not necessarily so. To illustrate this point, I'll use an example from my book on treating food allergy. Allergic illness can be compared to the water in a bucket. The bucket does not overflow until more water is added than it can hold. Likewise, allergic illness does not strike until the allergic person encounters more mites, molds, pollens, animal dander, fumes, and pollutants than they can tolerate.

Once the headache sufferer understands this principle, the way to treat the sick building syndrome becomes clear. Since they cannot change conditions in their workplace, and since they need to work to provide food and shelter, their only option is to reduce all the other allergic exposures in their lives. Once they do this, they will be more able to tolerate the exposure at work.

My nurses and I follow this principle as we battle the illnesses caused by the sick building syndrome. We urge our patients to correct those harmful exposures that are under their control—at home, at school, on vacation, and in their diet. By doing this, they may be able to live with the work exposures they cannot change. Most of the time, this is an effective measure and allows our patients to continue to work with some degree of comfort.

Jim's Story

Jim is a 36-year-old middle-level executive for a local high-technology manufacturing firm. His almost daily sinus and migraine headaches had responded well to our usual regimen of environmental changes, dietary avoidance, and allergy injections. He felt great when I saw him a year ago; however, his most recent visit was different.

Jan, one of my nurses, interviewed him before I spoke with him. He told her that his headaches had returned in full force, and they were definitely related to his work. His frustrating story unfolded as I talked with him later.

"Jim, Jan told me your headaches are back. Tell me about it," I prompted.

"They sure are, Dr. Walsh," he said. "I'm getting them at work. I'm okay on the weekends, but every day at work, about eleven o'clock, I feel really tired, my throat gets sore, and I feel a headache coming on. By two o'clock in the afternoon, it's so painful I can hardly stand it. It starts in the back of my neck, goes over the top of my head to my forehead, and then into my eyes."

"I am sorry to hear that, Jim," I said. And I was. I hate to think of my patients suffering such unbearable pains. "Has anything been done to find the cause?"

"Yes, the company had the building inspected, and they did a lot of work on the ventilation system. But it didn't help. I still have headaches, and so do a lot of the other people who work with me—many feel sick constantly."

"Is the company doing anything further to correct the problem?" I asked.

"No," Jim replied, with a sigh of exasperation. "In fact, they just circulated a memo saying that everyone knows that the cause of headaches is ninety-five percent psychological."

I was sorry to hear that last bit of news. Although anxiety and tension can have a major impact on headaches, I don't know any psychiatrist or psychologist who believes that headaches are ninety-five percent psychological. I did not doubt, though, that the owners of the company felt this way, especially after all their efforts to improve the work environment failed. Nor did I doubt that no further steps would be taken to find and correct the cause of this obvious case of sick building syndrome.

Although the environment where Jim works is the primary factor in his illness, he is not without fault himself. He has both a cat and a dog, and is taking no steps to limit his contact with them. In fact, he allows the cat to sleep on his bed. He also keeps far too many plants in his home and has restocked his aquarium with fish. He stretches the time between allergy shots to once a month, instead of getting them weekly, as his unfavorable environment demands. To add insult to injury, he indulges his sweet tooth by eating lots of refined sugar, and grabs a can of chili from the vending machine for lunch every day. I would be very surprised if the chili did not contain huge amounts of the food chemicals that cause headaches. Jim is definitely overloading his bucket of allergies.

The Meaning of Jim's Story

Jim's story is like a refresher course on the sick building syndrome. Look at all the points it raises:

- He experiences the typical symptoms of headaches, tiredness, and sore throat.

- His symptoms strike at work and disappear on weekends.

- His coworkers are also affected, many with recurrent upper respiratory infections.

- His company management recognizes the problem, but the subsequent inspection and building modifications are not effective.

- Jim is forced to continue working in the building.

- Management believes the symptoms are psychological and therefore not caused by conditions in the building.

- Jim does nothing to change the environmental and dietary factors under his control.

- Jim's headaches return in their former severity.

I don't know whether Jim will follow our advice and bring his home environment and diet under control. I haven't seen him since that last visit. I do know that—if he follows our recommendations—his chances of relieving these frequent and severe head pains are excellent.

* * *

If you carry any one thought away from our discussion of the sick building syndrome, I hope it is this: The sick building syndrome is treatable. But, just as charity begins at home, treatment of illnesses related to the workplace has to begin at home. This means following our suggestions and eliminating the moisture, mold, mites, and other home exposures that, when added to those you encounter at work, at school, or on vacation, make you sick. It also means taking your allergy injections more frequently and reducing or eliminating the foods and beverages that contribute to your headaches.

Since you can't always fight the sick building syndrome with a frontal assault, your best option is to attack this enemy with a rearguard action. One of the tactics that can be used in this battle is to avoid foods and beverages that may be contributing factors, which is the subject of the next chapter.

Foods and Beverages That Cause Headaches

Because I lived with severe headaches during my teens, I sympathize with other headache sufferers. I know first-hand how distracting it can be to live with pain so much of the time. I suppose that's why it is hard for me to believe these people are just chronic complainers, or are so emotionally crippled they need to conjure up imaginary head pain to hide their inadequacies.

As a fledgling allergist, I began to wonder whether the resources available in my specialty could help these people. I began to aggressively seek out patients with frequent and severe headaches, testing and treating them with moderate success. Certainly, our patients were grateful for the relief our treatment provided them—they had had little relief up until then. Their headaches tapered off—striking less often and less painfully. But they did not go away completely, and I was not satisfied. I felt I could do more.

Sue's Story

Sue, a student at one of our local colleges, is a case in point. We started her on a treatment plan, and when she returned to our office after the first three months, our conversation went something like this.

"How are you doing, Sue," I asked.

"Much better, Dr. Walsh," she replied, with the friendly smile that indicates a patient is happy with treatment. "I used to have headaches daily, and now I only get them twice a week and most hurt much less. I haven't had to miss school for the past month. And I'm only having one migraine every two weeks now."

I don't know how you would define successful treatment, but two headaches a week with two migraines a month did not spell success to me. In spite of our help, Sue was still missing out on a lot of study time because of her head pain—which couldn't help but have an effect on her grades. Why couldn't I do better? What was I missing?

The Missing Factor—The Diet

When the answer finally came to me, I felt like the person who finds his missing car keys locked inside the car—the most obvious place. The role the diet plays in allergy should have been obvious to me, but at that stage in my development as an allergist, my attention was focused on the environment in which my patients lived and worked. Thus I ignored what they ate and drank. My preconceived notion that food allergy played only a minor role in the headaches experienced by a few patients kept me from recognizing it played a major role in most cases. In retrospect, I could kick myself for not seeing what was right there in plain view the whole time.

The reason for the diet's importance should have been obvious—just as my patients with headaches were breathing in allergens from the environment, they were also ingesting them from what they ate and drank. Treating the mites, molds, pollens, and other allergens in the environment is essential for good headache control, but by itself, it is not enough. It won't correct headaches caused by foods and beverages. To treat them, the diet must be changed.

Changing the diet is a simple concept, but learning how to do it was not so simple. I should have realized that identifying the problem foods and beverages would not be easy. My patients are intelligent, and if pinpointing the dietary causes of their headaches had been easy, they could have done so without my help.

After years of searching, and with my patients' help, I finally identified these foods and beverages, and now that their identity is known, they can be avoided. When our patients avoid them, their headaches become less frequent and painful. They no longer need accept having two headaches a week as successful treatment.

Demystifying Food Allergy

Understanding and diagnosing food allergy is complicated by a phenomenon that is difficult to explain. Although it would be logical to assume there is only one type of food allergy, the fact is, there are two. I characterize them according to the reactions they cause—sudden or delayed—and the chart on the following page highlights their differences.

Sudden Food Allergy

This allergy strikes quickly after the offending food or beverage is ingested, usually within minutes. Those with sudden food allergy who eat a food they are sensitive to—shrimp, peanuts, nuts, fish, wheat, or other foods—quickly experience distress. The distress varies from person to person. It may include headaches, hives, wheezing, cramps, diarrhea, swelling in the throat, low blood pressure, and in severe cases, life-threatening choking or shock. The affected person is often very frightened, and for good reason—the symptoms can be dangerous.

Because these symptoms strike during or soon after a meal, it is easy to pinpoint the cause. Seldom does the afflicted person mistake the identity of the food or beverage that causes such rapidly developing and frightening illness.

The susceptible person usually reacts to only one or at most just a few foods. These foods are specific to that person, with few other people reacting to these same foods. For instance, Tom reacts with headaches from eating shrimp, Dick from walnuts, and Harry from eggs. Tom can eat walnuts and eggs without experiencing headaches, Dick can eat shrimp and eggs with no trouble, and Harry is not bothered by shrimp or walnuts.

Tom, Dick, and Harry do not need to eat large amounts of shrimp, walnuts, or eggs to react. A tiny bite—sometimes only a trace of the food contained in another dish—may set off a whopper of a headache. When the food hits their mouths, their bodies immediately identify an objectionable protein or carbohydrate found only in that food and quickly release a flood of histamine-like chemicals that precipitate cruel head pain.

There is only one treatment for sudden food allergy—avoidance. Tom, Dick, and Harry, and all others who are afflicted with this type of food allergy, must always avoid eating the foods that set off their sudden reactions.

Delayed Food Allergy

Where sudden food allergy is easy to detect, delayed food allergy is just the opposite. Sudden food allergy involves proteins and carbohydrates found in only one or a few foods, but delayed food allergy involves food acids, amino acids, and sugars found in many foods and beverages. Because numerous foods and beverages can cause the same symptoms, identifying which specific ones a patient is sensitive to can be very confusing.

Unlike sudden food allergy, which strikes quickly after even tiny amounts of offending foods are ingested, delayed food allergy waits until the sensitive person eats or drinks more of the offending food acids, amino acids, or sugar than he or she can tolerate. It can strike quickly if a single meal overloads this tolerance, or it may strike hours or even a day later if it takes several meals to overload the system. That's why Mary, who is nursing a headache with her morning coffee, doesn't even dream her pain is caused by the foods and beverages she consumed yesterday. She has no idea why she hurts.

SUDDEN AND DELAYED FOOD ALLERGY

Characteristics	Sudden	Delayed
Each patient has a different pattern of food allergy	Yes	No
Almost all patients react to the same foods	No	Yes
How quickly symptoms appear after eating	Minutes	Minutes, hours, days
Symptoms cause headaches	Yes	Yes
Food components responsible	Proteins and carbohydrates	Food acids, amino acids, and sugar
Patient identification of food	Easy	Difficult
Usual number of foods involved	One or a few	Many
Overload necessary before reaction occurs	No	Yes
Removal or reduction necessary	Removal	Reduction
Avoidance helps control headaches	Yes	Yes

Patients with delayed food allergy do not react every time they ingest these food chemicals—they can tolerate a small amount without pain. Thus, they may eat a food or drink a beverage on many occasions without experiencing headaches, as long as their tolerance is not overloaded. Because they suffer no consequences, they mistakenly believe the food or drink is harmless when it is not. If they do not realize that their headaches occur because they have eaten or drunk more of something than they can tolerate, they will be confused. They will have no way of knowing what is causing their pain.

To make things even more confusing, people with delayed allergy are often *primed* to react to combinations of food chemicals (sugar, food acids, amino acids) because the body does not clearly distinguish one from another. Therefore, if Mary eats a food with one of these chemicals (for instance, sugar), her body is primed to react to a meal or snack that contains the others (food acids or amino acids). Even though Mary did not overload on any one chemical, the combination of a slight excess of all three brings on her head pain.

Overload, priming, variable time of onset, multiple foods and beverages involved—these factors mask the identity of the foods and beverages that cause delayed food allergy. But all my patients with headaches share this allergy and must identify which foods and beverages they are sensitive to so they can avoid consuming more than they can tolerate. (I realize that *all* is perhaps too inclusive a term, but my experience in treating patients with headaches has taught me that few patients can ignore their diets without suffering pain.)

The more frequent and painful the headaches, the more carefully the diet must be restricted. If the headaches are less frequent and less painful, less restriction is required, and many patients with mild headaches can entirely disregard food allergy. However, today's mild headaches can turn into tomorrow's severe headaches, so even those with mild headaches should be aware of these foods and beverages—they may have to avoid them in the future. More severely affected patients have no such luxury. They must take immediate steps to avoid these foods today or they will suffer.

Food Allergy Is Not Difficult To Understand

I read every article about food allergy that I find in the medical literature. In essence, they all say basically the same things. Food allergy is difficult to understand, difficult to diagnose, and difficult to treat. I do not agree.

Recognizing that there are two types of food allergy dispels much of the mystery surrounding this condition. It becomes understandable, diagnosable, and very treatable. Yet it does not make it easy to treat. Three things are necessary for successful treatment of food allergy, and they relate specifically to delayed food allergy:

- Patients must believe it exists.

- They must know the identity of the offending chemicals and where they are found.

- They have to follow the diet.

The best way I know of to convince my patients that delayed food allergy exists is to describe how I first began to see evidence of it in my practice and my own reluctance to believe it can cause painful headaches. But the story of how I came to recognize and understand the connection between these seemingly harmless food chemicals and my patients' symptoms is a long one. Realizing that it would be impractical to repeat this story to each patient who came to see me, I began to entertain thoughts of writing a book.

As I began to write about headaches, I came to another realization. Teaching my patients about the environmental sources of headaches and about the relationship between headaches and food allergy was too big a task for one book. I decided I had to tackle food allergy first.

In *Treating Food Allergy—My Way*, I had four objectives in mind: (1) to help my patients understand the role of certain food chemicals in causing allergic illness, especially delayed food allergy; (2) to teach them to recognize the foods and beverages that cause their debilitating symptoms; (3) to describe the development of a diet to help them avoid harmful foods and beverages; and (4) to offer practical advice on following the diet in their everyday lives.

Does *Treating Food Allergy—My Way* accomplish these tasks? I think it does, because so many of my patients have commented favorably on its usefulness. The following conversation with Mary Ellen is typical of ones I have had with many patients since the book was published.

We were discussing Mary Ellen's headaches, which were responding nicely to allergy injections and diet changes, when she told me with a twinkle in her eyes, "I'm buying four of your books today, Dr. Walsh."

I could barely contain my pleasure as I replied, "That's nice, Mary Ellen. But why four books?"

"I lent the book to my mother in Arizona," she explained. "She was getting sick all the time, but since she's been following the diet, she's feeling much better. She wants a copy of her own, and she's going to send a copy to my uncle in Oregon for his birthday—he has migraine headaches. And I've shown the book to some people I work with, and two of them asked me to get copies for them."

Mary Ellen's story delights me and sometimes makes me envious of the book. My patients are always lending it to family and friends who live far from my office, and it has traveled to many more places than I have.

However, no matter where the book goes, if it helps someone, I am pleased. If you have frequent and painful headaches and want to learn more about the role of delayed food allergy in giving rise to them, please read it.

Following the Diet

For those with sudden food allergy, it is not difficult to eliminate desired foods and beverages from the diet. The symptoms that immediately follow even a small bite of the offending foods are extremely uncomfortable, often frightening, and sometimes dangerous. These painful symptoms quickly put an end to any cravings the person with sudden food allergy might have for these foods.

It is entirely different with delayed food allergy. My patients suffer headaches because they crave these foods and beverages, and giving them up is not easy. The reluctance to reduce or eliminate desired foods and beverages can often be a real barrier to treating delayed food allergy.

The patients who come to me for treatment are courageous. They refuse to accept the idea that their headaches are something they have to live with and are determined to do whatever is necessary to conquer these dreadful pains. Not one of them is happy to be told they must stop eating and drinking the foods and beverages they love, but very few lack the drive and determination to fight these cravings. For them, the barrier is not insurmountable.

You might be thinking that as a passive observer, it is easy for me to preach abstinence from the foods and beverages linked to delayed food allergy because these foods do not affect me. Nothing could be further from the truth. I must follow my own advice or suffer the unfortunate consequences. I share the same cravings my patients experience.

In fact, if there is a heaven, and if I happen to make it there some day, I often fantasize that St. Peter will meet me on the steps, not with a handshake, but with a huge platter heaped with all the foods and beverages I must avoid. And I will sit right down and eat every last morsel before I go in.

* * *

Treating headaches without changing the diet is like trying to compete in a cross country ski race wearing only one ski or trying to run a marathon in work boots. You can try it, but you probably won't get very far.

Part VI
Diagnosis and Treatment

Not All Allergists Agree

It is time to turn our attention to the allergist's office to examine the methods we use to diagnose and treat headaches. This is also an appropriate time to point out that the methods I use are not used by all allergists. In fact, many disagree with both my ideas and my methods. For some, even the suggestion that allergy causes headaches is a dubious one.

The Controversy

A recent conversation with members of my nursing staff gives evidence of this controversy. Jan, one of my nurses, was describing a telephone call she took from a patient who was considering coming to our office for the first time. "A friend had been trying to convince her to see us for treatment of her headaches," Jan related. "Before calling our office, she had phoned two other allergy clinics to ask if they thought her headaches were caused by allergy. Both said no. They told her that allergy rarely causes headaches."

Shirley, another of my nurses, joined the conversation. "I received a similar call this week and one last week. The callers had also spoken with several other allergists' offices and been told the same thing: 'Allergy doesn't cause headaches.'"

I was reminded of this conversation not long afterward as I listened to the following story told by a new patient.

Phil's Story

Phil is a computer analyst with a local company who suffers severe headaches in his forehead and temples, and this pain has been with him for the past three years. Medications give him little relief, so he convinced his doctor to send him to an allergist. I am acquainted with this allergist and know that he is an eminently qualified and highly respected physician.

He tested Phil, found him allergic to the house dust mite, and placed him on allergy injections for this sensitivity. After nine months of treatment, Phil still suffers from painful headaches. This apparent treatment failure must have renewed and confirmed my colleague's belief that, for the headache sufferer, allergy treatment is not the answer.

Wouldn't it be difficult for any knowledgeable observer to disagree?

No, not at all. Especially if the observer understood the causes of headache. He or she would ask Phil about his home and learn that he owns a ten-gallon aquarium and many plants; and that his finished basement is carpeted and contains stuffed furniture and many books. Through questioning, the observer would also learn that Phil uses a room in his basement for an office, that he spends much time there working on his computer, and that his headaches started soon after he moved his computer work to the office in his basement.

Further questioning would reveal that Phil's headaches peak during the spring and fall pollen seasons. Finally, his diet includes large amounts of the foods and beverages that cause headaches.

Having learned these facts, our hypothetical observer would have told Phil, as I did, "Phil, your headaches will be difficult to treat as long as you continue to be exposed to moisture, mites, and molds from your plants, your aquarium, and your finished basement. They may be impossible to treat as long as you use your basement office, which exposes you to more mold and dust mites than you can tolerate.

"Your diet should be changed to reduce or eliminate the food chemicals that cause headaches. In addition, we should pursue further skin testing to search for the pollen and mold allergies that your history suggests and add them to the house dust mite extract in your allergy injections.

"If you change your environment and diet, and we add mold and pollen to your allergy injections, we have an excellent chance of reducing or ending your headaches."

The Future

Phil's failure to respond to the treatment he received prior to seeing me does not condemn allergy treatment, but it does show the futility of inadequate allergy treatment. His story—similar to those of many other patients—highlights the problems allergists encounter in trying to treat headaches. Results will be poor if they treat only part of the cause. These poor results may explain why many allergists refuse to believe that allergy treatment of headaches has merit.

This distresses me and I know it distresses my nurses. We dislike being the subject of controversy. However, failing to provide our patients with effective pain relief is something we dislike even more. If we must be controversial to treat our patients, then so be it.

Each year we treat hundreds of patients with headaches of various types. Although some of our patients do not respond to treatment, most respond very well. If they reduce the moisture, mite, and mold levels of their homes, and if they follow our dietary advice, most of our patients live relatively free of pain. For those with daily migraines, the frequency changes to weekly or monthly. For those with weekly migraines, the frequency changes to monthly or they disappear entirely. For those with sinus and cluster headaches, the results are similar. They experience relief that no other treatment has provided.

As long as my nurses and I can provide this relief, we will continue to do so.

* * *

One of the secondary goals of this book is to try to put an end to controversy by helping doctors and patients learn our methods of treatment. In the following chapters, I will discuss the tools of the allergist—the patient history, the skin test, and allergy injections—and describe their use in the diagnosis and treatment of the headache patient. I will also point out how these measures must be modified to allow the diagnosis and treatment of headaches. This does not require abandoning our modern understanding of allergy and the immune system. It only requires us to look at both in a different but more logical light—one that guides us to effective relief for our patients who suffer head pain.

After all, relieving pain is our primary goal.

The Patient History

In the medical lexicon, the patient's history is the story he or she tells the doctor about the illness for which treatment is being sought. If the patient suffers from headaches, information disclosed in the history about when the headaches began, what they feel like, and what sets them off is invaluable to the doctor in diagnosing and treating them.

We have already discussed some of the information revealed by the history—how coexistent allergy illnesses suggest that headaches are also caused by allergy; the type of head pain brought on by sinus, migraine, and cluster headaches—and there is no need to repeat those discussions here. However, it is appropriate to examine some additional information that the history reveals.

This information is important because it provides the clue that head pain does not always spring from only one source. Just as two or more criminals may work together to rob a bank, two or more illnesses may work in combination to precipitate distressing head pain. As we look for the illnesses that produce headaches, we should be aware of the possibility that there are multiple causes. All of them must be treated to ensure our patients the best chance for pain relief.

Because they often have a multiplicity of causes, it is a mistake to think that treating allergy will stop all headaches. It is equally wrong to believe allergy cannot complicate headaches caused by other illnesses. We should not focus our attention only on tension and anxiety, or only on arthritis and injury to the neck, or on any of the other combined conditions that produce head pain. Since allergy can coexist with these other illnesses, if we miss its presence, we will fail to receive the pain relief we deserve. Because this point is important, we shall examine it closely.

Headaches Have Many Causes

Even though I am well aware that headaches have many causes, I find it valuable to periodically refresh my understanding of their many origins by participating in a series of headache seminars.

The seminars began as the result of a conversation I had with a colleague of mine who is a neurologist. We were each commenting on the number of patients with headaches who sought our help. More than half of my patients suffer headaches that strike weekly or more frequently, and his practice also includes a large percentage of patients with significant head pain.

These high percentages led us to wonder whether there might not be a fair amount of people in the community who would benefit from more information about headaches, so we decided to organize a seminar on this topic and see if anyone would attend. To make the seminars more valuable to the audience, we invited several other doctors to join us. Another neurologist, a psychologist, and an orthodontist agreed to participate, so we arranged for a room that would hold thirty people and advertised the seminar locally. At the appointed time, sixty people crowded into the room meant for thirty. It seemed that the community did indeed want to know more about headaches.

I gave my presentation on headaches caused by allergy and then listened to each of the other doctors as they discussed the spinal and muscle injuries, brain tumors and aneurysms, stresses and anxieties, and dental malformations and temporal-mandibular joint dysfunctions (TMJ syndrome) that also precipitate headaches. Hearing my fellow presenters discuss the breadth of conditions they treat in their fields served to remind me that head pain can have as many origins as an octopus has arms.

We presented subsequent seminars, each one more well attended than the last, and I found that listening again and again to these other specialists describe their treatment of headaches was time well spent. It helped keep me abreast of the latest treatment methods and medications, as well as broadening my perspective of the nonallergic causes of headaches.

The information presented at the seminars is reflected in the experiences of my patients. Many suffer allergic head pain complicated by TMJ syndrome, whiplash injury, arthritis of the spine, anxiety, and other conditions. These nonallergy-related conditions must be controlled by the primary doctor or the appropriate specialist to ensure adequate pain control.

Because headaches can have many origins, the following caution is appropriate:

> *Headaches arise from many causes. They should all be investigated and treated. Proper diagnosis begins in the office of the primary physician and continues in the offices of the neurologist and any other specialist he or she recommends. Only after these doctors have been consulted should the diagnosis of allergy be considered and an allergist consulted.*

The money spent on investigating headaches—including that spent on expensive tests such as CAT scans and MRIs—is never wasted. When a patient I treat has received a good evaluation, I am relieved.

The multiple sources of headaches warrant still another caution:

The diagnosis of a nonallergic cause of headache does not exclude the possibility of headaches being caused by allergy as well. Like a bully, allergy delights in attacking areas already weakened by other illnesses. Any patient's headaches may be influenced by both allergic and nonallergic conditions.

Sister Carolyn's Story

Examples that illustrate these cautions are as numerous in my practice as jelly beans in a jar. Since I started treating Sister Carolyn only recently, her story is fresh in my mind.

She is a delightful Catholic nun, a pleasant reminder of the fine women who taught me in grade school. Belonging to a more modern age, instead of wearing her habit to my office, she dresses in a conservative but pleasant outfit that befits her dignified and friendly manner.

But her headaches are neither dignified nor friendly. She suffers sinus headaches as frequently as three times a week, and migraine headaches strike at least once a week. And they hurt dreadfully. The pain has plagued her for years, and she came to us for treatment because a friend told her about our success in treating headaches.

When I asked Sister Carolyn to describe this pain, she told me, without any attempt to gain sympathy, "I have pain in several areas. I have arthritis of the spine and a degenerating vertebra in my lower spine, and the pain is here," she said, leaning forward and placing her hands on both sides of her lower back.

"Does it shoot up to your head?" I asked.

"No, it stays there," she replied, "but I have more arthritis and another degenerating vertebra in my neck that the doctors believe was caused by a whiplash injury from an auto accident. This pain centers on the two bumps in back of my head." As she said this, she leaned forward and placed her hands on the back of her head where the neck muscles attach to the skull.

"I've had this pain for four years now, and when it flares up, a trip to my chiropractor usually helps relieve it."

I was becoming convinced that this woman didn't need a hair shirt to live a life of discomfort. "Where are your other headaches?" I asked.

She leaned forward again, this time bracing her elbows on the arms of the chair and, with a weary gesture, placed her hands over her forehead, eyes, and cheeks. "I feel the pain here," she said.

Sister Carolyn's story underscores the cautions I gave above:

- Before considering allergy treatment, she had a thorough medical evaluation to find the nonallergic causes of her pain.

- Although a preceding whiplash injury and her present spinal arthritis brought her great pain, they did not preclude allergy from inducing further pain. Each of these causes—including allergy—must be treated to give her the best chance of living with less pain.

Although it is speculation on my part—and I did not ask Sister if it was so—I suspect that the doctors who evaluated her pain thought they had found the entire cause when they discovered the obviously damaged vertebrae. How human it is to be satisfied with finding a single reason and not inquire if perhaps a second reason exists, or maybe even a third. In Sister Carolyn's case, there *are* three reasons: arthritis, degenerating discs, and allergy. If she had not recognized all three reasons, and if she had not been determined to relieve her daily distress, I would never have been given the opportunity to help her.

To summarize, an essential part of taking the history includes asking a patient if they have asked their primary physician to evaluate the cause of their headaches and if they have obtained the consultations and tests he or she suggested. This should be done before an allergy consultation is considered.

A Misconception

People like Sister Carolyn can only be helped if allergy is kept in mind. Unfortunately, many are prevented from considering allergy by a misconception I encounter frequently. I often see patients with hives, asthma, hay fever, or other allergic illnesses who also have headaches. When I ask if it ever occurred to them that allergy might be a cause of their headaches, they reply, "No, I never even considered it. Besides, my headaches are due to sinus." Although the patient might think this answer excludes allergy, it doesn't. It doesn't even make sense.

To understand why, let's use the example of patients whose chronic sinus inflammation causes their headaches. Let's further restrict our example to patients whose primary doctors and any relevant specialists could find no reason other than sinus swelling for their headaches. No tumors. No chronic infections. No nasal malformations. So what's causing the recurring sinus headaches in these patients who so frequently accept "sinus" as a reason for their pain?

The sinus cavities are part of the body, the same way the hands and feet are part of the body. If your doctor told you that the cause of the pain you were having in your foot was "foot," or that the cause of your sore hand was "hand," would you ever go back to him? It is just as ridiculous to accept the explanation that the cause of your headaches is "sinus."

This diagnosis only tells you *where* the pain is located. The questions you need to ask are: "But why does it occur there? What is causing it?" Only when you ask *why* will you get started on the path to finding the cause, a path that leads to the diagnosis and treatment of allergy.

Ask the same questions if your doctor tells you that you have migraine or cluster headaches: "Why? What causes them?" If the cause is allergy, there is an answer.

Using the Patient History To Diagnose Allergy in Sinus, Migraine, and Cluster Headaches

How do I know when headaches are caused by allergy? How do I tell allergic headaches from other types?

You may feel that I have neglected to answer these questions. In fact, you may think I have avoided them to this point. If that is what you're thinking, you are right. But since we are discussing the history, the story told by the patient that allows the doctor to distinguish allergic headaches from other types of headache, the topic can't be avoided any longer. I have to admit the embarrassing truth. I don't know how to tell the difference.

My ignorance comes not from lack of experience—I treat several thousand patients with headaches. Nor does it come from a lack of training—I am a board-certified allergist. It comes from the fact that I do not believe I have ever met a patient with sinus, migraine, or cluster headaches who did not have allergy as a major cause or the only cause.

Now I realize that is a pretty controversial statement, and many doctors will have a difficult time believing it. But because I want you to consider that, just like hay fever, headaches are allergic reactions, I will tell you why I feel this way. Before I go any further, though, let me remind you of which headaches I am including in this discussion and which I am not.

The headaches I am referring to are those for which no cause has been found. This means that headaches caused by high blood pressure, tumors, aneurysms, diabetic hypoglycemia, strokes, arthritis, neck injury, TMJ, and any other medical condition that causes headaches are excluded. These conditions are not related to allergy. However, as I mentioned earlier, allergy can complicate these nonallergic illnesses, and to the extent that allergy is worsening the pain, it should be included in our discussion.

Why do I believe that, in the patients I see, headaches, like hay fever, are simply another manifestation of allergy? I have reached this conclusion by deriving it from the fact that headache patients respond to allergy treatment. My nurses and I treat hundreds of new patients with headaches each year, and rarely does our treatment fail to help them. If allergy is not causing their pain, why does this treatment work?

Could the reason for this excellent response to treatment be that we selectively treat only patients with allergic headaches? No, it couldn't. Our patients make the choice to come to see us, not the other way around. Any patient who comes to our office with distressing headaches is offered treatment.

Could it be that the opposite is true? Could patients with nonallergic headaches be avoiding our office? Yes, it's possible, but I see no evidence that this is so. Our office doors are open to anyone seeking our help.

Therefore, if it is true that my patients are a representative sample of people with headaches, then allergy is a major cause of headaches.

I have other reasons for believing that the typical sinus, migraine, or cluster headache is an allergic headache. One reason is the headaches that occur during the summer pollen seasons—they are unquestionably due to pollen allergy. Why else would they strike during peak pollen times? It also seems logical to me that if summer pollen causes head pains, the same headaches occurring in winter must be the result of the mites and mold that live in our homes in winter. Therefore, I believe that both summer and winter headaches are symptoms of allergy.

Still another reason is the allergic illnesses that so frequently accompany allergy. The coexistence of these symptoms points to allergy as the cause of headaches, a further indication that headaches are also symptoms of allergy.

If you can see some merit in these deductions, you may agree that patients (1) who have been adequately evaluated by their primary doctor and any other recommended specialists, (2) who have had appropriate treatment for any nonallergic disorders, and (3) who still suffer headaches should have the chance for adequate allergy evaluation and treatment.

Distinguishing Among Sinus, Migraine, and Cluster Headaches

We discussed how the location and type of pain determines whether we suffer from sinus, migraine, or cluster headaches. Because the patient history tells the doctor which type of headache bothers his patient, let's review this information again. As we do so, I will try to answer two questions: How do we distinguish one headache from another as we listen to the history? What difference does it make?

The answer to the first question—how we distinguish one headache from another—is easier to understand if we return to our explanation of how allergy causes headaches.

We postulated that all the illnesses of allergy arise from a swelling in the skin or somewhere inside the body. If the swelling involves the nose, it causes a stuffy nose. If the swelling involves the intestine, it stimulates diarrhea; in the skin, it causes the itch and redness of hives; in the air passages, the result is coughing, sore throat, and wheezing.

If the swelling occurs inside the inelastic sinus cavities, it causes the pressure ache called sinus headache, and if it develops around the blood vessels of the head, it causes the throbbing pain of migraine headache.

If the swelling surrounds the nerves that lie beneath the skin of the face and scalp, it causes perhaps the most devastating pain of all, a pain my patients find difficult to describe. They usually describe it by saying that it is neither pressure nor throbbing, but some other horrible type of pain. Because "nerve headache" does not seem an appropriate name (it sounds as if the patient is imagining the pain, and this pain is far from imagined), and for want of a better name, I lump it into the category of cluster headache.

Each headache reflects its origin. Sinus headache brings a pressure pain that is usually felt over the sinuses in the forehead, behind the eyes, and in the cheeks. To confuse us, it often jumps from these areas and appears elsewhere in the head, very commonly at the back of the neck, where it is mistaken for tension headache or pain caused by neck injury or arthritis.

Migraine headache also tries to confuse us by appearing wherever it wants to appear, but its presence is betrayed by its characteristic throbbing. It can be kind and cause only mild head pain, but it can also be cruel and frequently causes vicious pain.

Cluster headache also tries to conceal its identity by appearing in different places in different people, but it can be diagnosed because of the desperate pain it inflicts. Patients also frequently characterize it as a sharply localized pain. They can pinpoint the location of the pain it causes, which corresponds exactly to the network of nerves that lies on the skull. It frequently follows the network of nerves that begins below the eye and extends to the cheek, or the one that begins above the eye and travels to the eyebrow and forehead. At other times, it follows the network of nerves that passes over the temple or scalp.

This is an admittedly simplified way to distinguish these three types of headaches. It avoids having to make all the minute distinctions described in a neurology textbook, distinctions that are significant for the neurologist but less so for the allergist. Which brings us to the answer to our second question: What difference does it make to distinguish one headache from another?

As far as allergy treatment goes, it makes no difference at all. No matter where the swelling occurs—sinus cavity, blood vessel, or nerve—the treatment is the same. Measures that control or eliminate swelling in the sinus cavities also control swelling in the blood vessels and the nerves.

A Brutal Sharing—Ben's Story

Not only do sinus, migraine, and cluster headaches share the same cause, they share something else, as can be seen in Ben's story.

Ben is a single father of two delightful but rambunctious boys who accompanied him on his first visit to my office. Their busy play made the interview a challenge, but I didn't mind (Little Ben liked to sit on my lap), and Ben couldn't help bringing them. His babysitter was sick.

Ben told me his headaches were frequent and often very painful. Raising my voice to be heard above the clamor of little voices, I asked him to tell me where he felt the pain.

"It usually starts as a pressure pain in my forehead and in the back of my neck," he answered in an equally loud voice, placing one hand over his forehead and the other behind his neck. "If I take some aspirin right away, it often keeps the pain from getting worse. But sometimes I forget the aspirin, and other times the aspirin doesn't help. Then it gets worse and my temples start throbbing," he continued, shifting both hands to the sides of his head.

"Sometimes it gets even worse, and the pain travels up the back of my head and over the top into my forehead." Up to this point, Ben had used his whole hand to indicate where he felt pain. To describe this pain, however, he used only two fingers, drawing parallel lines that started on each side of the back of his head and traveled forward until they reached his forehead. He was drawing the path of the network of nerves that travels under his scalp.

What Ben was describing were headaches that began as moderately painful sinus headaches, transformed themselves into more painful migraine headaches, and completed their transformation by becoming severely painful cluster headaches.

Often, as Ben's headaches slowly dissipated, they reversed this progression—cluster headaches became migraine headaches, which became sinus headaches—and finally disappeared like an ice cube melts into water and then evaporates.

Besides being caused by the same swelling, what do sinus, migraine, and cluster headaches share? They share Ben.

Is Ben's Story Unusual?

Unfortunately, no. It is one that is frequently told by the patients I treat. Their suffering reveals the characteristics of all three types of headaches. As in Ben's case, many patients experience sinus headaches followed by migraine headaches, which often peak as cluster headaches, each succeeding headache more painful than the last.

There can be only one conclusion. In allergic people, the three types of headaches doctors spend so much time and energy identifying are simply different stages of the same headache. Realizing this simplifies the task of understanding why the same allergy treatment suppresses all three.

* * *

The patient history—the story patients tell a doctor about their headaches—contains extremely useful clues to the identity and causes of this pain. It separates headaches into sinus, migraine, and cluster headaches, or combinations of all three.

The history also provides hints as to whether headaches are caused by allergic or nonallergic conditions. Often it points to more than one cause. It guides the doctor in deciding which diagnostic tests to use and which treatments are appropriate.

All the doctor has to do is listen.

The Allergy Skin Test

Whenever I think about the allergy skin test, I am reminded of a story a good friend told me. A clever little toy that changed from a warrior hero to a car, a plane, or a tiny army tank was quite popular at the time, and my friend Jerry was fascinated by it. He spent a great deal of time one afternoon standing at a toy counter, trying to get one of them to work. He even enlisted the help of the toy salesman, but no matter how they twisted and tugged, those two overgrown children couldn't seem to figure it out.

Just as they were conceding defeat, a little boy walked up, holding onto his mother's hand. He was so small, Jerry and the salesman had to lean way over the counter just to get a look at his face. With the mother's permission, they handed the toy to the little guy and asked if he could make it work.

Gripping his pacifier firmly between his teeth, the child turned the toy over several times to study it, then set to work. Pulling one way and twisting the other, his hands moving so quickly they were almost a blur, he transformed the warrior into a car in the blink of an eye. Without a word, he handed the toy back to the two chagrined adults, then turned and marched off, once again clinging to his mother's hand.

"Bill," Jerry lamented to me later, "you haven't known true humiliation until you've had to ask for help from a child with a pacifier."

Jerry's story not only makes me chuckle, it also has a moral. Sometimes, in spite of all our intellectual twisting and pulling, a problem is so confounding it resists even our most valiant attempts at understanding it. Then, conceding defeat, we must seek the help of a child. That's what happened to me when I first tried to understand the allergy skin test.

Stevie's Story

The event I refer to happened many years ago, long before I received my allergy training at the Mayo Clinic. At the time, I was a general medical doctor in the Air Force, and since there was no allergist on the base, I was responsible for the skin testing and allergy treatment. One of my patients was Stevie, a little boy with severe asthma.

Although I had only a rudimentary understanding of allergy at the time, I was convinced Stevie's asthma was caused by allergy, but I could not prove it. On several occasions, I skin tested Stevie, and each time the tests showed nothing. No allergy to ragweed. No allergy to dust. No allergy to cats and pollen. No allergy to anything.

A short time later, Stevie became very ill with asthma and I had to hospitalize him. For some reason (it's been so long I can't remember why), I decided to repeat the skin tests after he had been hospitalized for a week, and asked permission from his parents, who kindly agreed to let me do them.

The results flabbergasted me. In the previous testing, house dust had produced not even the tiniest hive. This time, the hive around the house dust sample was as fat and red as a cherry tomato. The row of molds, which had also produced no reaction in the earlier tests, now glowed like a string of garish red Christmas lights. The skin surrounding the ragweed area erupted in a hive as soon as the droplet was placed on his back.

What Does It Mean?

Stevie's skin tests made no sense. I relied on them to make the diagnosis of allergy, but in Stevie's case, they were both confirming and denying this diagnosis. One day they showed no allergy, another day they showed flagrant allergy.

What if your x-ray showed you had a malignant tumor one day and none the next? What if your blood sugar test showed you had diabetes one day and not the next? Would you trust these tests? Of course not. You would disregard them because they would be obviously wrong and useless.

Shouldn't the same be true for the allergy skin test? Yes, it should—with one exception. The test would have value, and we would be grateful for its help, if the blame for these inconsistent and unreliable results lay not in the test itself, but in how we interpret it. This is an important point, because the diagnosis of allergy depends on a positive skin test. Yet, with headaches, the skin test often shows no allergy. These negative results seem to deny that allergy has any role in causing headaches.

This seeming contradiction leaves us with two alternatives: either allergy does not cause headaches, or it does and we are misinterpreting what the test is saying. I believe the latter is true.

To better understand what the test is trying to say, we must return to our discussion of the immune system, because the skin test is trying to tell us something about this important system.

The Immune Army

A system as complicated as the immune system can be looked at in several ways, each very accurate but each also presenting a somewhat different viewpoint. In our earlier discussion, we compared the immune system to an army swimming in the bloodstream. To understand what the skin test reveals about the immune system, I find it helpful to move our army onto dry land and think of it as an army defending a city.

Present-day military weapons and tactics are so sophisticated that using a modern army for our example might complicate our discussion. Instead let's use a medieval army, one that fights with armor and swords, on horseback and on foot.

The city our army defends is fortified by forbidding stone walls and a mammoth central castle built to resist a siege. Surrounding the city, as far as the eye can see, are verdant fields that produce a bounty of food for the inhabitants and a surplus of grains for export. The city shines with beauty and prosperity.

But there is a price to be paid. Just as the city's wealth nurtures its inhabitants, it also attracts its enemies. They are many, they are strong, and they are constantly attacking. Not a month goes by without small marauding bands or large armies marching through its broad and inviting valleys, bent on looting and plundering the city's treasure.

Still, these would-be conquerors find no easy victory. A disciplined and ferocious army awaits them. Protecting the farms and approaches to the city are legions of light cavalry, armed with sword and pike and mounted on swift horses. Called the Emergency Response Divisions (E divisions), they destroy the small bands and delay the large armies, giving the city precious time to prepare for battle.

When the enemy forces are numerous and skilled—and their onslaught relentless—they exhaust the E divisions and break through to march on the city. Nearing the gates, they find they must face the defenders of the wall. More heavily armed than the E divisions, the Guard and Mobilization Divisions (G and M divisions) are trained to meet these attacking forces and crush them.

But they do not always crush them. A ferocious attack mounted by overwhelming numbers of enemy soldiers can overcome even the stalwart G and M divisions and gain entrance to the heart of the city. But even this inner core is not left defenseless. The invading army is now met with the most heavily armed, most skilled and determined of the city's defenses, the Lance divisions (L divisions). Like knights of old, the L divisions annihilate the enemy force before it can taste the sweet wine of victory.

The city survives, not because its enemies suddenly become peaceful or no longer covet its riches. It survives because its defenses are both fearsome and layered in depth—rapidly responding, lightly armed E divisions, supported by slower responding, more heavily armed G and M divisions, and finally, by the firmly entrenched, most heavily armed L divisions.

The City and You

Your body is like this city. Deadly germs find you an irresistible prize. Germs that cause brain infections called meningitis, lung infections called pneumonia, bloodstream infections called septicemia surround you and are constantly on the attack. Each would like to claim you as a morbid trophy, but you survive in spite of their unending assaults. The valiant knights in your immune army savagely defend you. They do not let you die.

As in the city of our example, not only are your defenses fierce, they are also layered in depth. But they are not divisions of soldiers, but hordes of antibodies (proteins specifically made to attack germs). The fast-moving and wide-ranging E divisions represent the E antibodies (called immunoglobulin E or IgE) that fight the germs trying to gain entrance to your body. The slower and more heavily armed G and M divisions represent the G and M antibodies (IgG and IgM) that fight off the germs that manage to gain entrance into the body. The slower and more heavily armed

L divisions represent the potent lymphocytes that respond to infection slowly but devastatingly.

What Do IgE, IgG, IgM, and Lymphocytes Have To Do With Skin Tests?

Everything. They are what the skin test measures.

As we learned earlier, the same immune system that protects you from deadly germs also makes your life miserable. Not only are the IgG, IgM, IgE antibodies, and lymphocytes primed to attack germs, they are also primed to attack harmless allergens like dust mites, pollen, mold, animal dander, and food. (Remember, an *allergen* is the part of pollen, dust, mold, food, etc., that causes allergy.)

Although we all possess these immune cells that are primed to fight allergens, some of us never show any allergic symptoms. No hay fever, no stuffy nose, no abdominal cramps and diarrhea. The suppressor lymphocyte stops the immune system from bringing on these illnesses. In other people, this cell fails at its task, releasing the illnesses of allergy. (I am one of these unfortunate souls.)

The skin test gives the allergist a peek at those antibodies and lymphocytes that are dedicated to fighting pollen, dust mites, mold, animal dander, and food. To explain this, I'll describe what happens when Arleen, one of our allergy nurses, applies the skin test to your skin.

The Prick Test

Three separate skin tests measure antibodies and lymphocytes. To perform the first, the prick test, Arleen uses a dropper to apply a drop of fluid to your skin. Dissolved in this fluid is a tiny amount of ragweed pollen, prepared by a company that specializes in making allergy tests and solutions.

Where does this company obtain the ragweed pollen? From a person who vacuums the pollen from a ragweed plant as it pollinates in the fall. (Imagine trying to explain to your prospective mother-in-law that you make your living vacuuming plants.)

Back to Arleen and the test. After applying the drop of solution, she lightly pricks the skin, allowing a small amount of dissolved ragweed into the top layer of skin, where the IgE antibodies cluster. If the drop finds an IgE antibody that specializes in fighting ragweed, it stimulates this antibody, causing it to release a flood of histamine underneath the drop. The histamine quickly swells the skin into a hive and turns the nearby skin an angry red. This hive and redness signals to Arleen that the test is positive.

Arleen continues the drop and prick procedure using other dissolved pollens as well as dissolved house dust mites, animal dander, molds, and foods. Sometimes the positive tests show both a hive and redness, at other times they show only redness. As with the ragweed test, each positive response signals the presence of IgE antibodies that specialize in fighting the allergen she is testing.

The Intradermal Skin Test

Although your history may point to ragweed pollen and other allergens as the cause of your stuffiness and headaches, the prick test often doesn't. There is no redness and no swelling. Then Arleen must proceed to the next test, in which she injects some of these same test materials into the top layer of your skin. The amount she injects is so tiny it looks smaller than the swelling from a mosquito bite.

This injection acts like an invading germ entering the body through the skin, calling forth the IgG and IgM antibodies that patrol the bloodstream, poised to attack ragweed pollen or other allergens. If these antibodies are present, redness and swelling signals a positive test.

The Delayed Skin Test

Once again, although your history may point unerringly to ragweed and other allergens, the prick and intradermal skin tests may not. For instance, you may experience miserable headaches during the fall ragweed pollen season, but your ragweed skin test doesn't even blush pink.

Don't worry yet. There is still another test—one that seeks out lymphocytes that are committed to fighting ragweed (and hurting your head as they fight). To find these lymphocytes, Arleen performs another skin injection, again using dissolved ragweed pollen. This time she increases the strength of the pollen in the injection solution and injects an increased amount, so the total dose of pollen injected is a lot larger than the dose she used in the preceding intradermal test.

Why the increased strength and dosage in this test? Because the lymphocyte takes so much time to stir itself and drag itself slowly to the test site. Enough ragweed pollen must be injected to prevent the body from removing it from the test site before this slowpoke cell arrives.

Because of the slowness of the lymphocyte reaction, we cannot read the test in the same twenty minutes that we read the rapidly reacting prick and intradermal tests. You have to return to the office the next day for us to see the results.

And not only does this test take longer, it is also harder to read. There may be only a faint redness in a strongly positive test. Of more importance than the redness is something a doctor learns to feel with his fingers after long experience—a firm bump that arises beneath the test site. This bump signals a positive test.

Since the result takes overnight to develop and we do not see you during this time, we ask you to look at the injection sites at the sixth hour after the test is applied. This is because, occasionally, one or more injection sites will flare at the sixth hour. This flare is caused by the late arrival of IgG and IgM antibodies. Sometimes, the flare will last until we read the test the next day, but at other times the swelling and redness will disappear by the time you return to the office. If you spotted it at the sixth hour, we can recognize the test as positive.

A Warning

The allergy skin test can cause dangerous reactions and should only be performed by an adequately trained nurse or physician who is aware of these dangers. The above description of the test is not meant to instruct a doctor or layman in how to apply the test, but is simply an attempt to tell the reader what happens during the test. The above information is not enough to permit anyone to perform skin tests.

Does the Skin Test Diagnose the Cause of Today's Headaches?

Doctors use many tests to diagnose illness. X-rays are used to diagnose lung tumors, blood sugar tests to diagnose diabetes, and the skin test to diagnose allergies.

But, does the skin test tell us why your head hurts today? At first, the answer would seem to be "Of course!"; however, on second thought, maybe that answer is wrong. If you have been trying to follow this strange logic, you should be unsure of the true answer.

In solving the mystery of what the skin test measures, we can turn to no better advice than that of Arthur Conan Doyle's Sherlock Holmes: "It is an old maxim of mine that when you have excluded the impossible, whatever remains, however improbable, must be the truth."

To follow his advice and arrive at the true answer, let's first discuss the qualities that a test to diagnose the cause of today's illness must possess:

- It must be unchanging, either positive or negative, but never both.

- It must always point to the correct cause.

In both of these cases, the allergy skin test flunks.

You know from Stevie's story that his allergy skin test reacted strongly negative one day and just as strongly positive another day. In fact, that pattern repeated itself—in retests, it reacted positively when he was hospitalized and negatively when he was not. Therefore, the allergy skin test is not unchangeable; it can be both positive and negative in the same person.

Does it always point to the correct cause? Absolutely not. We see many patients who sneeze and wheeze all through the fall ragweed pollen season but experience neither of these symptoms in the spring tree pollen season. Yet, their tree pollen prick test flares the same angry red as their ragweed pollen test. We also see many patients who suffer tree pollen congestion and headaches in the spring but who have no miseries whatsoever in the fall. Their ragweed pollen test is an identical twin to their tree pollen test, falsely diagnosing fall pollen allergy. The skin test is diagnosing pollen allergy that does not exist.

If the skin test diagnosed allergy, why would a positive test say patients suffer from hay fever during seasons when they are free of symptoms? Further, why would it lie about the large number of patients with identical hay fever and headache stories whose prick and intradermal skin tests are absolutely negative? They are as allergic to pollen as patients with positive tests. Yet the test falsely says they are not.

To further confound the believer in the diagnostic usefulness of the skin test, it often confidently diagnoses allergy—by its positive reactions—in people who have never suffered an allergic reaction in their lives. How could anyone believe this test correctly diagnoses allergy?

Therefore, the allergy skin test does not always point to the correct diagnosis. In fact, it often denies the correct diagnosis.

Obviously, this is a crummy test on which to base a diagnosis.

Would you allow a doctor to cut into your chest to remove a tumor diagnosed by an x-ray you could not trust? Would you base your decision to use insulin on a blood sugar test you could not rely on? No, you would not.

Closing in on What the Test Is Trying To Tell Us

Let's return to the celebrated detective's advice. We have excluded the impossible—the test is not trying to tell us why our patients are suffering symptoms today. Then, what is it trying to tell us that makes it so valuable doctors still use this test decades after it was first discovered? Thankfully, there are clues to help us find the true answer. We already know that:

- The prick test measures the allergen-fighting IgE antibody.

- The intradermal and six-hour delayed tests measure the allergen-fighting IgG and IgM antibodies.

- The twenty-four-hour test measures allergen-fighting lymphocytes.

- Nonallergic people react positively to the test.

- The test depends on the environment (hospital versus home, in Stevie's case).

When Sherlock Holmes explains to Dr. Watson why the improbable answers are the true answers, he removes the mystery and the answers become not only probable but also indisputable. Although I feel that I am being overly ambitious—like the fly trying to steal the sugar bowl—I will also try to resolve our mystery. So wish me luck and buckle your seat belts.

The most important clue was provided by Stevie (the *Stevie Principle*?). First of all, Stevie was allergic. The large positive reactions to house dust, mold, pollen, and animal dander that erupted on his skin test in the hospital proved this. Then did the skin test lie about this allergy when he was out of the hospital?

No, it didn't, and to understand why, let's return to our city under siege. Under continuous, heavy assault by a horde of determined enemy forces, the E, G, and M divisions became exhausted. If an observer tried to find them in our medieval city, they would be gone. He might then leap to the following conclusion: Since the city has no E, G, or M divisions, it must not need them. Only a city that was permanently at peace would have no need for these divisions. Therefore, the city must be permanently at peace.

You, being aware of what was really happening, would be amazed that anyone could reach such a mistaken conclusion. "Can't you see what's right in front of your eyes?" you ask. "The city walls lie in ruins. The houses are burning. The citizens are dying. The L division is fighting an implacable enemy that is crowding the streets. Don't you understand that the E, G, and M divisions are absent, not because they are unnecessary, but because they are exhausted."

Then, in the kindly tone and carefully measured speech you reserve for those of lesser ability, you say, "This city is not at peace. It is under constant attack."

The same is true for Stevie. When he was at home, the mite and mold content of his musty home constantly assaulted his immune system, exhausting his IgE, IgG, and IgM antibodies. They could not signal his allergy to the inquiring skin test. In the filtered air of the hospital, removed from these high mold and mite exposures, these antibodies recovered and profusely responded to the test.

If an observer leaped to the conclusion that Stevie's asthma was not allergic because his skin test was negative, he would be mistaken. Stevie's test was negative, not because he was *free* of allergy, but because he was *overwhelmed* by allergy. Stevie was under such heavy bombardment from allergens that his asthma was dreadful, exhausting his IgE, IgG, and IgM antibodies and keeping them from reacting to his skin test.

So the test never lied. It was simply that his immune army was unable to respond.

Stevie's Not Alone

Am I not drawing a wild conclusion from one experience with one patient? I don't think so.

Let's look at the incident itself. Of the multitude of patients with allergic asthma, isn't it more likely that Stevie's case is typical, instead of some peculiar deviation from normal? In other words, if ninety out of a hundred patients had typical allergic asthma, isn't it more likely that Stevie represents the ninety percent than the ten percent?

Doctors recognize that any particular illness is more likely to be caused by the usual causes than those that are rare. That's what is meant by the old adage, "When you hear hoofbeats, think of horses and not zebras." (In some parts of Africa, they probably think of zebras and not horses.)

Besides, being of a religious frame of mind, I think that our divine guide sometimes presents us with an unexpected lesson in truth, and we must learn from it, especially when the lesson involves a child.

Turning from Stevie to the other patients we treat, we see ample evidence of skin test suppression. We see patients with headaches during the pollen seasons who have negative prick and intradermal tests to pollen. Their headaches disappear with allergy injections tailored to fight the effects of pollen.

We see patients with headaches who live in musty houses and apartments. Their mite and mold tests are blank. Correcting the home problems and using mite and mold allergy injections controls their headaches.

If we were not aware that the skin test can be suppressed, and if we thought a negative test meant the absence of allergy, these miserable patients would have no option but to continue to suffer. We would not have treated them, and that would be a shame.

It Is Important To Do All Three Tests

In the patients I just mentioned, the skin test is not completely negative. Although the prick and intradermal tests measuring IgE, IgG, and IgM antibodies are frequently suppressed by overwhelming exposure to pollen, molds, and house dust mites, the delayed test is not. The lymphocyte seems highly resistant to environmental suppression and will give a positive test when the antibodies do not.

This is a great help. It helps our patients who desire some proof of their allergies before accepting our recommendations for treatment, especially before agreeing to allergy injection treatment. It is also a great help to my nurses and me. We find good evidence of the activity of lymphocytes committed to fighting mites, molds, and pollens. The positive delayed test helps direct our treatment.

The negative prick and intradermal tests also help. They tell us we must look for overwhelming mite and mold exposure when our patient's tests are negative.

The delayed test for lymphocyte allergy is seldom used by other allergists. Many use only the prick test for IgE antibodies, believing that the absence of IgE antibodies directed against ragweed pollen or other allergen means no sensitivity to these allergens. Others use both prick and intradermal tests to measure IgG and IgM as well as IgE. If these are negative, they test no further.

They do not test for the last member of the immune army, the lymphocyte. Why? I do not know. Would you search your house for a child's lost ball, and not finding it, refuse to also search the yard? Would you search for a job in your city and, not finding one, refuse to also look for one in the suburbs? No, in both cases you would call the search incomplete until you finished it.

How can you search the immune system for allergies and ignore the lymphocyte?

What the Skin Is Trying To Tell Us

At last we come to the final clue that explains the mystery—what is the skin test trying to say? In stories of Sherlock Holmes, this is the time when Sherlock enlightens a mystified Dr. Watson. Even though my profession is the same as the perpetually perplexed Dr. Watson—and it is presumptuous for me to try—I will try to end the mystery by playing not Watson but Holmes.

The final clue to the skin test arises from the fact that people free of allergy may show positive skin tests. This not only proves that the skin test is not trying to tell us the cause of today's headache, but it also hints at what it is trying to say.

It measures the ability of a person to have allergy, whether this allergy is causing today's headaches, will cause headaches tomorrow, or caused headaches in the past. It measures this ability only if the antibodies and lymphocytes are capable of responding. It measures the *basic status of the immune system.*

A *positive* skin tests does not say, "This patient is sick today because she is reacting to ragweed pollen and house dust mites." It simply says, "This patient has antibodies and lymphocytes able to react against ragweed pollen and house dust mite. I cannot tell you if she is reacting to them now, reacted in the past, will react in the future, or perhaps will never react to them. However, I can tell you that, at this time, they are present and have not been overwhelmed."

A *negative* skin test tells a different story. Everyone has antibodies dedicated to fighting allergens such as mites and ragweed pollen. In the patient with headaches, when the tests do not show these antibodies on the prick and intradermal tests, they signify that the antibodies have been overwhelmed by the environment and are not there to react. Then, only the delayed test still functions because it measures the hard-to-dominate lymphocytes. These cells are still fighting. In other words, the tests are reporting: "Status—IgE, IgG, and IgM down for the count. Lymphocytes still fighting."

The Suppressor Lymphocyte

Although antibodies and lymphocytes dedicated to fighting ragweed pollen and a host of other harmless allergens are present in all of us, they cannot fight if the suppressor lymphocyte makes them stop. When this cell is strong, there are no allergic symptoms. When it fails, allergic illnesses arise because the immune system runs out of control, causing congestion, headaches, and other miseries.

Unfortunately, the skin test does not report the status of this important cell. If it could, this information, together with the information it gives about the rest of the immune system, would allow the test to diagnose the cause of today's headaches.

One Little Complication

If I have explained the skin test adequately, you will realize it is a simple test, easy to understand. But, as with so many other simple things, there is one extra bit of information that complicates it.

So far we have been describing the test as if all allergic patients were identical, but of course, they are not. Just as there are two ways to react to food allergens, there are also two ways to react to environmental allergens such as mold, pollen, dust mites, and animal dander.

One of these occurs in people who produce huge amounts of IgE antibodies sensitized to ragweed pollen, house dust mites, and the other allergens. These people show huge positive results when they are skin tested. When they have allergy symptoms, they suffer striking illnesses.

They sneeze, they wheeze, their eyes water, their skin itches when they are exposed to the allergen that causes their discomfort. If it is ragweed pollen, they look miserable during the height of the ragweed pollen season. If it is tree pollen, they sneeze or wheeze in the spring tree pollen season; if it is cats, they break out in hives when they hold cats; if it is wheat, they wheeze when they eat wheat. If they react to a combination of allergens—which is often the case—they spend most of year feeling miserable.

There is a second way for patients to react to environmental exposures. This occurs in allergic patients who do not produce huge amounts of IgE antibodies. Their prick test results are not dramatic, nor are their symptoms dramatic. They suffer repeated colds, chronic nasal stuffiness, persistent wheezing, diffuse aches and pains, or any combination of these symptoms, plus other ongoing illnesses.

What difference does it make whether people with headaches produce large or small amounts of IgE? Those with high IgE production are more likely to be diagnosed as allergic and treated with allergy medication and injections. Their obviously positive reactions to prick and intradermal tests help them find treatment.

People who do not have large amounts of IgE are less likely to be so diagnosed. They are also less likely to be treated than people with high IgE.

Are people with high and low levels of IgE similar? Yes. Both are allergic and both feel miserable because of their allergy. Both can suffer from headaches. Also, in my experience, both can have their skin tests suppressed by overwhelming exposure, especially to house dust mites and mold. If this happens, the dramatic symptoms of the high IgE producers can fade and be replaced by the same chronic and persistent pain and discomfort suffered by those who are not high IgE producers.

Why would two types of allergy exist? I don't know, but I believe that the high IgE producers possess an unfortunate gene that allows far more IgE production than a wise nature should permit. Then, if the suppressor lymphocyte fails, they are condemned to woeful discomfort.

Allergic patients who are not high IgE producers are more of a mystery. Why should they suffer? I believe there is one answer that satisfies the clues that surround them. They should never have been allergic in the first place.

They suffer because they are stuck in an environment with such high levels of allergens that their immune system crumbles. They are normal people who unfortunately live in a musty home.

Cleaning Up Some Odds and Ends

You may be guessing that some doctors believe only in the prick test because they believe in only one type of allergy—the allergy that happens to the high IgE producers. That would be my guess as well.

You may be concerned about the allergic people who do not produce large amounts of IgE—who treats them? They concern me as well.

* * *

Why Was This Chapter So Long?

The skin test is often used to diagnose the cause of today's illness. The test does not do that. The negative prick and intradermal skin tests seem to deny that allergy causes headaches. The test does not do that either.

Some day you may be skin tested and the prick and intradermal tests may show no positive reactions. You may then be told that these results prove your headaches are not caused by allergy. I believe that is a wrong interpretation of the tests, and I wanted you to know why I feel this way.

The chapter had to be long enough for me to explain that.

Allergy Injection Treatment

In a perfect world, how different things would be. Over-weight people would be slim and frail people sturdy. All adults would be charming and witty, all children respectful and obedient. And quiet.

And no one would live in a musty home.

The Nelsons' Story

Linda brought eight-year-old Roger and ten-year-old Julie to see me recently. Both shared the same painful headaches, a combination of sinus pressure and migraine's throb with a suggestion of cluster headache's localized pain. Both suffered from these pains frequently; the annoying headaches occurred daily, the severely painful headaches twice a week. They lived a wretched life.

Their primary doctor had pursued a very competent and complete evaluation, including a CAT scan, but had uncovered no reason for their headaches. A pediatric neurology exam was scheduled at the university hospital, and the children had already been evaluated by an ENT surgeon. Linda told me, "He looked in Roger and Julie's noses

207

and said they were allergic. I decided to bring them to see you."

I was pleased that the children had received such an excellent evaluation before coming to see me. But I was not pleased when I learned the cause of their headaches.

Shirley, one of our nurses, had already taken a detailed history, including a diet and environmental history. Their diet included the foods and beverages that cause headaches in our patients. The environmental history was even worse. The Nelsons lived in a very old house that they had gutted and restored—"It's like new now," Linda told me proudly. But in all the renovation, the basement had remained untouched.

Only one-fourth of the house extended over the basement; the remainder rested on a concrete slab or over a dirt crawl space. The dirt crawl space was vented, not to the cleansing outdoor air, but directly into the basement. I have no idea how many molds, yeasts, and algae flowed into the basement from this crawl space. I also did not know what life forms flourished in the carpets lying on the cement slab in the old basement.

Linda reacted to my concern with the assurance: "But we never go into the basement."

I felt sorry for her. Linda's effort to change an old musty house into a healthy home had been well-meaning but misguided. It hadn't worked. I replied, "I'm glad you don't use the basement, because if you did, Roger and Julie would be much worse. But even upstairs, they breathe basement air. Even though you don't go down into the basement, the basement air comes upstairs."

The treatment for Roger and Julie's headaches was obvious. In a perfect world, the Nelsons need only move to a newer and dryer home and the children's pain would subside.

But the Nelsons cannot move. The old house was the only house they could afford. The cost of the renovation plus the mortgage payments absolutely prohibited a move to another home. They were stuck there.

The Reason for Allergy Injections

The Nelsons are not the only family that lives in such surroundings. Nor are they the only family that has tried to change their surroundings by gutting the house while ignoring the basement. They also are not the only family that cannot move.

But all is not hopeless. Given enough time and a reduction of their debt, they can eventually move. Or they can find some way to convert a musty basement with high levels of mites, mold, yeast, and algae into a dry basement with low levels of these organisms.

Other families with similar problems can also correct them. Perhaps the basement is not the major source of their problems. They can find a way to vent the home if it is too tightly insulated or repair the moldy wall caused by rain or snow penetrating the wall and rotting the insulation. But while they make these changes, they need effective treatment to control their headaches.

Fortunately, treatment is available. The diet can be changed to reduce or eliminate the foods and beverages that aggravate their headaches. The impact of the mite, mold, pollen, and animal dander in the air they breathe can be counteracted by allergy injection treatment.

What Is Allergy Injection Treatment?

Remember Arleen's skin test? She used dissolved pollens, molds, foods, animal danders, and house dust mites to prompt the immune system to react, reading this reaction as positive if she saw swelling or redness. We use the same dissolved allergens in allergy injection solutions (called extracts because they are extracted from pollens, house dust mites, etc.). These extracts are used, not to stimulate the immune system, but to quiet it.

Doesn't make much sense, does it? Our patients—burdened by excessive mites, molds, pollens, and animal danders—come to us for help, and we treat them by injecting more of the same allergens that are causing their pain. Isn't that like feeding sugar to diabetics, or fat to the overweight?

Not really. For some reason, proven years ago, the way an allergen gains entrance to the body determines how the immune system reacts to it. For instance, if ragweed pollen is blown into a ragweed-sensitive person's nose, the person becomes painfully allergic to the ragweed, a condition called *priming*. Priming is more than a laboratory curiosity. It happens in real life every fall to ragweed sufferers. The more days of ragweed exposure, the more severe the sneezing and wheezing until, at the end of the season, the affected person is far more miserable than at the start.

Contrast that with what happens when ragweed pollen, instead of being blown into the nose, is injected under the skin. The immune cells become less active. They get sleepy. Now, when the hay fever sufferer breathes ragweed pollen, the immune system provokes far less sneezing and tearing. The allergy sufferer has achieved a state of *tolerance*. Perhaps not a state of perfect tolerance, but far better than the hyperallergic state existing before the injections.

We see the same effect with allergy injections using other pollens, molds, animal danders, and house dust mites. In the patient with headaches, injections rob these allergens of much of their pain-generating power. Comfort replaces the pain. For the patient living in a musty home, the relief is a godsend.

Does the Immune System Stop Fighting Germs?

Do treated patients become tolerant not only to harmless allergens, but also to the harmful germs that cause pneumonia and septicemia? Do they lose their protection against infection? No, they don't.

Like the well-trained German shepherd allows its sight-impaired master to safely cross dangerous streets, the allergy injection allows the immune system to tolerate only the pollen, mold, mite, and animal dander allergen contained in the extract. The germ defenses are completely unaffected, and as before, patients fight infections effectively.

The *tolerance* conferred by allergy injections differs from the *immunization* produced by tetanus, measles, and other immunizing injections. Immunizing injections awaken sleeping immune defenses so they will be strong and active if the injected germ tries to attack. In allergy, the immune defenses against harmless allergens are already too strong. Allergy injections dampen these hyperactive defenses, bringing them back under control.

Do Allergy Injections Work?

Yes, they do, a fact that has been well proven. Studies with *ragweed* pollen show beyond a shadow of a doubt that ragweed pollen injections calm the severe sneezing and congestion of the fall hay fever sufferer. Similar studies show valuable symptom control with *other pollens* (i.e., grass pollen), *house dust mite, cat dander, and stinging insect venom.*

Studies of *mold* allergy injections return inconclusive results, not because they are ineffective, but because evaluating the results is complicated. For instance, patients living in homes with moldy basements breathe various types of mold plus yeast, algae, and house dust mite. In these patients, a scientific study may involve giving injections of one of the molds encountered in the basement. Evaluating these injections is difficult because, even if they worked well, the symptom relief would be obscured because the patients would still be reacting to the other microscopic inhabitants of this airborne zoo. The results are inconclusive, which makes for some very frustrated scientists.

In our practice, allergy injections containing combined mold, yeast, and algae control headaches so well that I believe they are very helpful.

Food shots are almost universally condemned by allergists. However, some hints are appearing in the allergy literature that in the right patients, they are effective in relieving food allergy.

I suspect that when allergists understand the two types of food allergy, sudden and delayed, food injections will overcome their bad reputation. I believe they will be found to be helpful for patients with *sudden* food allergy. I also believe that only avoidance—not food injections—will help patients with *delayed* food allergy.

How Allergy Injections Work

The immune response to allergy injections is complicated, but for our purposes, there is no need to delve deeply into these complexities. Reviewing their effect on lymphocytes and antibodies adequately shows what the injections do.

The *IgE antibodies* (the antibodies measured by the prick test and responsible for the misery of allergic illnesses like hay fever and hives) are profoundly affected. We will confine our attention to those delinquent IgE antibodies that make a career of fighting a pollen such as ragweed. Any decrease in these antibodies helps the IgE overproducers who suffer such uncomfortable sneezing, itching, headaches, and wheezing from this troublesome antibody. Surprisingly, injections cause an increase in this antibody rather than a decrease.

Fortunately, this increase only lasts through the early part of injection treatment. After that, the IgE levels remain steady for a time, then later undergo a slow decline.

An even more significant event occurs during the hay fever pollen seasons. If the hay fever sufferer does not receive pollen injections, each pollen season stimulates a sharp increase in the production of pollen-fighting IgE antibodies. But if the patient receives pollen injections, the rise in IgE levels is aborted. The IgE levels do not increase during the pollen season. This is a blessing, because this rise in IgE levels almost certainly contributes to the increasing misery of the hay fever sufferer as the season advances

Because there is no seasonal increase in pollen-fighting IgE levels, and because continuing injections are depressing these levels, the affected person enters the next pollen season with fewer antibodies to cause symptoms. This helps explain why patients on pollen injections experience increased comfort during the second and subsequent years of treatment.

Although the IgE antibody's response to injections is well known, the effect on *IgG* and *IgM* antibodies is still not fully understood.

What happens to the *lymphocyte?* Quite a bit, actually. When ragweed pollen and other allergens enter the body, the lymphocytes that fight these allergens divide and multiply wildly. (We have already discussed how allergens gain entrance to the body.) Allergy injections slow this multiplication like fire retardant slows the spread of a forest fire. Fewer allergen-fighting lymphocytes mean less misery.

This reduction in unwanted lymphocytes provides evidence that the weakened suppressor lymphocyte is gaining strength. It is becoming more active, telling the immune system to stop this senseless fight against the harmless allergen. Because a weak suppressor lymphocyte causes allergy, strengthening it allows injection treatment to directly fight the allergic state. It does not just mask symptoms. It is the only treatment able to do this.

Finally, remember the *mast cells* (and their cousins the basophils)? They release the histamine that causes so much allergic misery. These cells are also affected by allergy injections. Before treatment, contact with a tiny amount of an allergen such as ragweed forces the mast cell to discharge its stored histamine and cause miserable symptoms. After injection treatment, the mast cell's release of histamine changes. Far more ragweed is required to stimulate this cell, and not all its histamine is released when it is stimulated. In other words, the cell becomes more tolerant of ragweed. It becomes dormant instead of hyperexcited.

The effect of allergy injections on antibodies, lymphocytes, and basophils profoundly changes the immune system, soothing it and allowing the allergic person a measure of peace.

How We Give Allergy Injections

We give them very carefully. A patient may suffer severe and sometimes dangerous reactions to this treatment. Therefore, we start with a tiny dose that we believe our patient will tolerate and slowly increase the strength of the injection, allowing the patient time to get used to each stronger dose. For an example of this treatment, I'll describe how Corrine—one of our nurses—begins treating a typical patient with headaches.

Our patient, Mary, suffers frequent sinus and migraine headaches, and medications have given her disappointing relief. After completing her skin tests, I offer her the option of allergy injection treatments, and she decides to take them. To determine the strength of the starting dose, I review the intensity of the reactions she showed on her skin test. She had large reactions, so I decide to start her injections at a weaker strength than we usually use and mark this starting dose on her chart.

Corrine rechecks the skin test to see if she agrees with the starting dose. If she believes the dose is too strong for Mary, we review her chart together, and treatment does not begin until both of us are satisfied that the dose should prove safe. Injecting more allergen than Mary will tolerate is dangerous. A review of this dose by a registered nurse specializing in allergy treatment gives Mary an extra measure of security.

Once we agree on the dosage, Corrine prepares a schedule of gradually increasing doses of extract, and explains the schedule to Mary. She also warns Mary to watch for any reactions to the injections. Two types of reactions are possible, one annoying and one dangerous:

- The annoying reaction is a *local reaction*. As the name implies, it develops locally, in the area where the injection is given. Usually it starts hours after the injection and appears as a warm swelling that can be as small as a quarter or so large it affects the entire upper arm. Although irritating, this reaction is not dangerous.

- The dangerous reaction is called a *systemic reaction*. As its name implies, it reaches beyond the arm to affect a major system of the body. For instance, if it affects the respiratory system, it causes sneezing, wheezing, or other respiratory symptoms. If it affects the vascular system, it may cause the blood vessels to dilate, producing a drop in blood pressure.

The danger in the systemic reaction arises from the possibility of a patient's air passages becoming so swollen that breathing is blocked and the patient chokes. Or, the blood pressure may fall so catastrophically that a patient goes into shock. Since most of these alarming reactions start soon after the injection is given, we caution our patients to remain in the doctor's office for twenty minutes after an injection and report any suspicious symptoms.

If Mary is receiving her injection treatments at her primary doctor's office (as most of our patients do), we ask her to report any reactions to her doctor. We also ask her to call us and tell us about the reaction before she receives her next injection. Frequently, a reaction prompts us to modify her schedule, usually by decreasing the dosage or slowing the rate of increase, or both.

Certain events increase the chances of a reaction:

- Overproducers of IgE are more likely to react system-ically to shots than are patients with low IgE.

- Certain viral infections (colds) increase the chances of local or systemic reactions.

- People who live in musty homes often suffer local reactions at low doses.

My nurses and I carefully check the starting dose of the IgE overproducers—those whose prick test reactions are strongly positive—to make sure we start them on a low dose. As I mentioned, they can react systemically to doses that the low IgE producers take without complications.

Viral infections cause the allergic patient uncomfortable symptoms, including wheezing, hives, headaches, and more. They also complicate injection treatment. For instance, our patients may take injections for months with-out a hint of trouble, but then they suddenly and unexpect-edly experience local or systemic reactions. Because many of our patients experience problems at the same time, we know a virus is moving through the community, infecting our patients and causing them to react to their injections.

A regrettable but helpful hint that a patient lives in a musty home sometimes shows up during allergy injection treatment when they react to a low dose. Usually the reac-tion is manifested as a tender, warm swelling around the injection site. This swelling at a low dose is the body's way of saying, "I live with too much mite and mold to take these shots well." If the patient cannot eliminate this expo-sure, he or she often must accept a lower dose of injections than people living in dry homes.

Maintenance Injections

After taking progressively stronger injections for sev-eral months, patients reach the strongest dose we will use in treatment. This dose is called the maintenance dose. Not all patients reach the same maintenance dose. Some experience a local or systemic reaction at a weak dose and must accept a weaker maintenance dose that they can tolerate without trouble.

Patients receive this maintenance dose every week or so during the first year of treatment. The soothing effect of the injection lasts from five to fourteen days. When it wears off, their headaches and other allergy symptoms return. This return of symptoms signals the need for the next maintenance injection.

After the first year of treatment, some patients can stretch the interval between injections to three or even four weeks. In my experience, the length of time between injections depends on the environment. The worse the environment, the more frequently the injections need to be given.

A Warning

Allergy injection treatment can cause dangerous reactions and should only be performed by an adequately trained doctor or nurse who is aware of these dangers. The above description of this treatment is not meant to instruct a doctor, nurse, or layman in how to use injections. It is simply an attempt to tell the reader what happens during treatment. The above information is not sufficient to permit anyone to perform allergy injection treatment.

Is There Danger in Using Allergy Injections?

Yes, there is. That's why they must be used carefully.

The danger is the possibility of that most horrible of events—the death of the patient. This can occur when an injection reaction spins out of control and reaches a peak from which the patient cannot recover. That's why we try to be so careful in designing an injection schedule tailored to what we believe the patient can tolerate.

But danger is relative. A productive life would be impossible if we refused to accept the dangers we face each day. We could die from drowning on a fishing trip, from choking on a piece of food, or from slipping in the bathtub. These dangers do not keep us from fishing, eating, or bathing. We accept the risks because the danger is small. The question we must answer is: How dangerous are allergy injections?

This risk is hard to determine precisely because a fatal reaction from injection reactions is so rare. An event that occurs rarely is much harder to study than one that occurs frequently. Studies in the allergy literature indicate that there are from one to four fatal reactions per year in the United States from either skin testing or injection treatment. To simplify our calculations, let's say four people a year die of treatment.

Approximately ten million allergy injections are given each year. Therefore, the chance of any single injection resulting in a fatal reaction is about one in two and a half million.

Is this an unacceptable risk? Will we face less risk if we replace injection treatment with modern and potent headache medicines or the old standard pills used for years? These medicines also subject patients to risk—that of a fatal drug reaction. Often patients use two or more medications to control headaches, and each medication, even those as familiar as aspirin and antihistamines, increases the chance of a fatal drug reaction. In fact, if you could find any medicine that carries no risk of a fatal reaction you would have found a rare gem of a medicine indeed.

Therefore, replacing injection treatment with medicines does not eliminate the risk of a fatal reaction. Would avoiding both injections and medicines end all risk? Probably not. Suffering untreated head pain also carries a risk.

How many fatal car accidents involve a driver distracted by head pain? And how many fatal industrial accidents involve workers distracted by head pain? There is no way to know for sure how many of these fatalities can be attributed to headaches, but activities such as driving or using machines are dangerous at any time and must be considerably more dangerous when the operator suffers from untreated pain.

Making Injection Treatment Safer

Since injection treatment carries dangers, allergists strive to reduce this danger. They pay special attention to circumstances that increase the possibility of systemic reactions because these carry the greatest risk. These circumstances include:

- Rapidly increasing dosage schedules;
- Highly sensitive patients;
- Injections taken during a pollen season;
- Unstable asthma;
- Use of beta-blocker medications;
- The beginning of treatment (patients who have been undergoing injection treatment for some time have fewer reactions).

We use this information to reduce the chances of a systemic reaction. We try not to increase the dosage too rapidly. We need to be particularly careful if a patient is highly sensitive (large positive skin tests) and to be especially cautious when starting injection treatment in a new patient. We try to use injections with more caution when a patient has asthma and while giving pollen injections during a pollen season. We also ask the primary doctor to change beta-blocker medicines to non-beta blockers (ask your doctor if you are taking this type of medicine).

In our office, we try to reduce this danger even further by selecting maintenance doses that are not the very highest a patient can tolerate. There is always some guesswork involved in determining this dose, but I feel most comfortable erring on the side of caution.

* * *

We have barely scratched the surface of the subject of allergy injections. A full description of this treatment would easily fill a whole book. Because the subject is so complex, our nurses spend the first two years in our office becoming familiar with the techniques of using them. I know I cannot make you as knowledgeable as they are, but I have tried to briefly cover certain important aspects of this treatment.

I hope that you have become more familiar with allergy injections, how they work, and what dangers surround their use. I also hope I have made you aware of the steps a doctor takes to minimize these dangers. If so, I have accomplished the purpose for which this chapter was intended.

Is this treatment worthwhile? You bet it is. Who should use it? Let's look at that subject more closely in the next chapter.

Who Should Receive Allergy Injection Treatment?

I feel like a mother who tells the babysitter what to feed the children and when to bathe them, and then leaves the home without specifying when the children should go to bed. The information the mother gave the babysitter was incomplete. I wonder if I have given you incomplete information. I have told you about allergy injections, but have I adequately explained who should use them?

In a perfect world, no one would need allergy injection treatment. Changing the diet and environment would cure most headaches. However, the world is not perfect, and as we discussed earlier, although people with headaches can change their diet, their ability to change their environment is limited.

Hence the need for the allergy injections that attack the allergens in the home, school, and workplace—a treatment that works, not by covering up symptoms, but by soothing the overreacting immune system. But who should receive this treatment?

To answer this question, we should discuss the weaknesses and strengths of allergy injections. Once we know these weaknesses and strengths, we can assess their value and determine when to use them.

What Are the Weaknesses of Allergy Injections?

Can allergy injections permanently cure headaches? If they could, they would only be needed for awhile, and when they were stopped, the headaches would never return. This doesn't happen. Many of our patients continue injections for years because they need them; their headaches return unless the injections are continued.

Why do injections lack the power to cure? Because they cannot change the predisposition to allergy carried in the headache sufferer's genes. Injections also cannot correct the environmental exposures and diet factors that breed head pain, and correcting the environment and diet is the only true cure for allergic headaches.

Furthermore, injections cannot prevent all the headaches a patient suffers. During some viral infections or during times of peak allergen exposure—or when a patient departs too far from our diet—painful headaches still return in spite of this treatment.

Finally, injection treatments are inconvenient. In the life of a busy mother or office worker, minutes are precious and hours golden, and these treatments are time consuming. It is bothersome to have to go to the doctor's office, wait for the injection, wait for twenty minutes afterward, and then return to work, home, or school.

Then Why Are They Used?

With all these drawbacks, why would anyone ever choose to undergo allergy injection treatment? The answer is that it has strengths that other treatments cannot match.

It fights headaches for as long as patients need its help. The treatment fails only when a patient's environment is so full of allergens or the diet contains so many problem foods and beverages that its efficacy is blocked. With a reasonable environment and diet, it works well. The injections never lose their potency; the patient never becomes immune to their effects. Such consistent and potent help is unique to this treatment.

Allergy injection treatment reduces the frequency of headaches from daily or weekly to biweekly or monthly. It reduces throbbing pain to mild discomfort.

For those who fail to benefit from any other treatment, including the most modern headache medications, these strengths are impressive. Their lives have been dominated by frequent, painful sinus and migraine headaches, or by excruciating cluster headaches, or combinations of these headaches. Injection treatment soothes this pain. For these people, injection treatment is far less of an inconvenience than the pain it replaces.

While it is tempting to argue that taking medication up to four times a day is more convenient than injection treatments, not everyone would agree. For some, remembering a weekly appointment for an injection is easier than remembering to take daily medication. And once a patient has been on treatments for some time, going for an injection every two weeks or once a month is no more inconvenient than having a prescription filled. Many of my patients choose to forego daily medications and rely on allergy injections, which stop their headaches before they start.

Finally, allergy injections have one last advantage over any other treatment. Brad's story illustrates the importance of this advantage better than anything I might say.

Brad's Story

Brad is a middle-aged electrician who was sent to see me by his primary doctor because for years he has suffered from daily sinus and weekly migraine headaches. He has lived in almost constant pain. Brad's primary doctor had searched long and hard for a cause of his headaches, and finding none, suspected allergy.

Jan, one of our nurses, questioned Brad and found that he lived in a musty house, and although he suspected his musty house caused his headaches, he could not afford to move to a better home. In addition, his job forced him to work in dusty old buildings, and although he knew the conditions there bothered him, he feared leaving his job. The economy was tight, electrician jobs were scarce, and he was no longer young. He was stuck in a home and a job that caused his headaches.

Brad's skin test showed allergy to mites, mold, pollen, and food. He agreed to change his diet, but because diet changes could not fight his home and job exposures, we discussed allergy injections. "I would like to take them," he decided.

Curious as to why he chose the injections, I asked him, "Brad, I agree with your choice, but tell me your reasons for wanting this treatment."

"Because I am tired of headaches, tired of continually feeling sick, and tired of being tired," he replied with a heavy sigh. "I've tried all the headache medicines, and they work poorly for me. The ones that help the headaches don't stop the continuous colds and sore throats, and they don't make me feel any better. I have to go to work in spite of how I feel because I've already used too many sick days. If I miss more work days, I'll lose my job."

What His Story Means

Brad's reasons for wanting injection treatment are not unusual. Allergy involves the same immune system that fights germs, and when your body fights germs, you feel sick, tired, and often depressed. These feelings are a normal consequence of the frenetic activity of the hyperactive germ-fighting mast cells, lymphocytes, and antibodies as they attack germs or allergens.

Sickness, fatigue, and depression are a regrettable but necessary evil in your body's fight against illnesses like pneumonia or septicemia—you accept these symptoms because they are necessary to getting better. But they are not acceptable when your misguided immune system is fighting the effects of allergens. Not only are these symptoms unacceptable, they are also unending. Unlike with the immune system's fight against germs—which ends when the germ is defeated—allergic people never stop battling the pollens, mites, and molds that surround them every day of their lives. They continually feel ill and tired.

This constant battle saps their vigor; it intrudes on their family life; it interferes with and threatens their schooling or employment. It causes painful headaches.

In Brad's case, medication to blunt his headache pain gave him poor relief. His persistent illness and tiredness remained. Brad chose allergy injections because they fight both his headaches and his chronic fatigue.

Not all patients with headaches experience tiredness and recurrent colds and illnesses, but enough do to make this combination of headaches and illness one of the most common reasons for choosing allergy injection treatment.

A List of Reasons for Taking Allergy Injections

To summarize, my patients usually decide to take allergy injections if:

- Their headaches are frequent and painful:
  - They have episodes of cluster headache;
  - They have migraine headaches more than once a month.
  - They have sinus headaches more than once a week.
- Their headaches are accompanied by other allergic illnesses, such as:
  - Severe summer pollen hay fever;
  - Recurrent upper respiratory illnesses;
  - Other allergic symptoms—persistent cough, sore throats, hives, chronic rashes, eczema, asthma, nasal stuffiness.
- Medication provides little relief.

HEADACHES ARE FREQUENT AND PAINFUL. Because cluster headache brings such devastating pain, patients desperately seek relief. They readily accept injection treatment. Migraine pain, although severe, does not approach the intensity of cluster pain. Therefore, patients are more hesitant to use this inconvenient treatment unless the migraines occur more often than monthly. Sinus headaches, although also painful, usually do not hurt as much as migraine or cluster headaches. Patients will usually opt for injections if the pain occurs at least weekly.

These are only rough guidelines. Some patients seem able to tolerate excruciating pain, while others suffer tremendously from what often appears to be less severe pain. Those who suffer the most deserve treatment.

When patients experience mixed headaches (most of my patients do), their reasons for treatment do not fall neatly into these guidelines.

THE HEADACHES ARE ACCOMPANIED BY OTHER ALLERGIC ILLNESSES. A patient who must suffer other aggravating and tiring allergic illnesses along with headaches is more likely to desire injection treatment. Brad expressed this desire. He wanted treatment for more than just his headaches.

Patients with severe summer hay fever, chronic sore throat, chronic allergic rashes, chronic coughs, and other irritating and exasperating allergy symptoms share Brad's desire to both alleviate their pain plus enjoy freedom from feeling tired and sick all the time. They readily accept injection treatment.

MEDICATIONS PROVIDE LITTLE RELIEF. Finally, I am surprised by how frequently medications have given my patients inadequate pain relief. Many of the patients who come to us for evaluation are experiencing poor pain control from medications. Hopefully, from our discussion of allergic headaches, you can begin to see why.

Allergic headaches are caused by an out-of-control immune system whose mast cells, antibodies, and lymphocytes are frantically fighting the mites, mold, and pollens in our homes, schools, and workplaces. When the exposure is heavy, when the headaches are painful and frequent, when the patient suffers miserably, then medications can lose their ability to subdue symptoms. Allergy injections that strike at the wellspring from which these headaches flow can give patients the comfort they are in such need of.

Chosen versus Dictated

I always leave the decision of whether or not to use allergy injection treatment up to my patients. Why don't I make this decision for them? For a reason I think is very important.

Although I have had a fair amount of psychological training in medical school, and during my internship and residency, I possess no mystic ability to reach into my patients' minds. If I could, I would know how much pain and distress they have, and I could determine how far we should pursue treatment. Headaches leave no visible signs that a doctor can use to determine how much pain a patient is experiencing. Only the headache sufferer knows if the pain is severe enough and frequent enough to warrant the use of allergy injections. I cannot decide if my patients need treatment. Only they can make this decision.

* * *

If you are like me, you are fascinated by things that work well. Whether it's one of those new electric screwdrivers or a favorite old hammer, a sophisticated food processor or a reliable stain remover—they work for you. Allergy injection treatment works well, and I have been fascinated by it since I first started using it.

In this chapter, I have tried to present a balanced view of allergy injection treatment, comparing its strengths and weaknesses. But if anything I have said seems biased in favor of this treatment, it is because I am so impressed with its tremendous power to meet headaches head on and conquer them.

What other treatment has the ability to seek out and find the malfunctioning lymphocytes, antibodies, and mast cells in the allergic immune system? What other treatment can put a stop to their hyperactive attack on harmless allergens, thereby soothing the headaches caused by this senseless assault? What other treatment can do all these things while preserving the germ-fighting immune activity so necessary to life? There is no other treatment that possesses this power.

Therefore, in my admittedly biased view, when should you use allergy injection treatment? To put it as simply as possible:

- If you suffer painful sinus, migraine, or cluster headaches,

- And if they strike more frequently than once or twice a month,

- Or if you suffer milder headaches more frequently,

- And you cannot stop your headaches by changing your home, work, or school environment,

- Or by changing your diet,

- Why wouldn't you use this truly effective treatment?

Medications for Headaches

Treating headaches is like pulling dandelions. If you only pull out the top of the plants, they'll grow back. The root must be destroyed to get rid of this pesky weed.

Headaches are the dandelions in my patients' lives. Pain-reducing medications are a great blessing; however, like pulling out the top of a dandelion, they only work temporarily. To have more than a temporary effect, the roots from which headaches spring must be eliminated.

Sometimes head pain is rooted in arthritis of the spine, temporomandibular joint problems, whiplash injury, or similar causes. These conditions must be diagnosed and treated or there will be no lasting impact on head pain.

If headaches arise from the environment and diet, these conditions must also be diagnosed and treated or the headaches will reappear as surely as leaving the roots of the dandelion intact allows it to rise anew from the earth.

These thoughts guide my nurses and me as we treat our patients. We must destroy the roots that nourish headaches by investigating and treating allergy. This is our job. This is what brings patients to our office for treatment.

Because our patients' referring primary physicians or neurologists are well qualified to provide headache medications, I do not prescribe these medicines. Patients suffering from painful headaches should consult their primary doctor or neurologist to learn about the potent medications available by prescription in the modern pharmacy. We will not discuss them here.

Many medicines, including antihistamines and pain medications, are available without prescription, and if they help, patients with headaches should use these medicines. Since they are so readily available, it is appropriate to discuss them here. We also will discuss the use of cortisone medications because, used properly, they provide great pain relief.

Antihistamines and Decongestants

Whenever people think of medicine for allergy, they think of antihistamines and decongestants. As we learned when we explored hay fever, these medications help the hay fever sufferer and reduce the itch and redness of hives. Are they as useful in treating headaches? Unfortunately, they are not.

Antihistamines and decongestants combat the effects of histamine released from the mast cell by the IgE antibody. They calm the sneezing of hay fever and the itching of hives—at least the sneezing and itching caused by histamine. However, they do not slow the IgG and IgM antibodies, nor do they soothe the lymphocyte.

For our patients with headaches, histamine often contributes little or nothing to the pain of headaches. If it contributed significantly, patients with headaches would show large positive reactions to the prick skin test. (This test measures histamine and IgE response to allergens.) Usually, they do not; however, they often show large delayed reactions to antigens (the test that measures lymphocytes), indicating that lymphocytes are involved in headache pain.

Because antihistamines and decongestants have little effect on lymphocytes, they would not be expected to provide good headache relief.

I don't mean they shouldn't be tried. They are readily available and moderately safe medications. If used early in a headache attack, they may help. They may be especially useful in combatting headaches that accompany spring, summer, and fall hay fever.

Ask your local pharmacist for help in selecting these medications. Newer antihistamines that cause less sedation are available by prescription—Seldane® is one that acts quickly and may help. When using antihistamines and decongestants, follow the instructions given with the medicine, and do not use them if they are contraindicated for you.

Aspirin and Other Nonprescription Pain Medication

These are excellent medications for mild to moderate head pain. They are limited in their effect on severely painful headaches, which can be calmed only with far more potent and often addicting medications.

Aspirin not only decreases pain, it also reduces inflammation (the swelling that causes head pain). From what my patients tell me, aspirin and similar pain killers must be used quickly when headaches strike. Their soothing action is often defeated by any delay in taking them.

Be sure to follow the directions given with these pain medications and do not use them if they are contraindicated for you.

Cortisone or Steroid Medications

There are various forms of cortisone or steroid medications (the steroids used in treating allergy are not the same steroids used by some people for body building). These medications can be given in various ways, including by injection, in pill form, and in the form of nasal or oral sprays. We will discuss only those forms helpful in treating headaches.

Unlike antihistamines and decongestants, cortisone pills are a potent pacifier of the lymphocyte. Cortisone's ability to calm the lymphocyte at the same time it soothes headaches points to a close tie between this cell and sinus, migraine, and cluster headaches. How it does this is a topic too lengthy to discuss here.

I prescribe cortisone pills frequently because they stop headache pain. Rarely do they fail. However, they must be used with caution, the same caution a hunter would use in handling a loaded rifle, because if used carelessly, cortisone medications can injure a patient. Patients should carefully follow the doctor's directions.

To reduce the chances of harmful effects, oral cortisone treatment for headaches should be used:

- Only for severe pain;
- Only once a day, if possible (8:00 A.M. is best);
- In the smallest dose that works;
- For the shortest time possible.

Cortisone pills are not suitable for the treatment of mild headaches. Patients are better served by tolerating mild pain than by taking this potent medicine. However, when pain is tormenting and disabling, they are useful.

They are also unsuitable for patients who are just starting allergy treatment. Most of our new patients suffer such frequent and severe headaches that they would soon be injured by using too much cortisone. Unfortunately, living with frequent pain is less harmful for most patients than using too much cortisone.

In most cases, though, once allergy treatment has reduced persistent, severe headaches to rare occurrences, oral cortisone can be helpful, and the chance of overusing this medication diminishes considerably.

Cortisone is especially useful for patients whose headaches suddenly and unexpectedly recur after having responded well to treatment. I suspect that these returning headaches, which can last for days or weeks, are caused by viral infections. Cortisone allows us to regain—in just hours to a few days—the pain control that was disrupted when the headaches returned. Because our patients have become accustomed to living without the pain that used to plague them, these returning headaches can be especially cruel and the soothing effects of cortisone especially welcome.

I prescribe a form of cortisone pills called prednisone in a moderate dose, twenty milligrams, once a day. Used for one to five days, the pills usually stop the headache episode. Some of our patients suffer further recurrences of these severe headaches, and these recurrences are widely separated, less than once a month. When I see this pattern of recurring headaches developing, I give my patients a small supply of cortisone with the instructions to take one tablet as soon as they recognize the onset of another severe headache. Taken early enough, one tablet often aborts the headache, saving the patient days of terrible head pain.

Of course, this treatment is unworkable if the headaches are caused by too much moisture, mites, and mold in the home, or are due to a patient's refusal to eliminate offending foods and beverages from their diet. In such cases, the patient must learn to destroy the environmental and dietary roots of the headaches and not rely on cortisone. Cortisone has no place in these situations.

Cortisone Sprays

Our modern medicine chest contains cortisone specifically developed for use in nasal sprays. If used according to directions, little cortisone is absorbed from the nose into the body, which is both an advantage and disadvantage of using this form of cortisone.

Because the spray works at the surface of the lining of the nose, the cortisone's action is concentrated where it does the most good. In some patients, relieving nasal congestion by using these sprays prevents headaches.

Since little cortisone is absorbed from the nose into the body when used as directed, these sprays cause little or none of the harm possible with the use of oral cortisone. This is an advantage.

However, limiting the effect to the lining of the nose is also a weakness. Because so little cortisone is absorbed into the body, it cannot penetrate the closed and aching sinuses, as cortisone from pills does. It also cannot reach the swelling around the distant blood vessels and nerves of the head that causes painful migraine and cluster headaches. This is a major disadvantage compared to cortisone pills, whose effects reach the blocked sinuses as well as the blood vessels and nerves of the head.

Cortisone nasal sprays are certainly worth a try for people with headaches. They may be the answer for mild to moderate headaches, and they may calm some of the more severe headaches.

Cortisone nasal sprays are available by prescription only, so ask your doctor about them.

* * *

I have discussed these medications so that you can appreciate their usefulness in treating headaches. If and when you use them, follow the instructions printed on the label of the nonprescription drugs, and follow your doctor's orders if you use prescription drugs. Do not use them if you have a medical condition that prohibits their use.

Antihistamines, decongestants, and aspirin-like pain medicines allow you to treat your own headaches without the bother of obtaining a doctor's prescription. Each is readily available in pharmacies and can help treat mild and infrequent headaches.

However, do not let the availability of self-treatment blind you to the wisdom of consulting a physician. Remember that headaches can be caused by life-threatening conditions such as high blood pressure, tumors, and aneurysms that require medical diagnosis and treatment. They can also be caused by chronic medical conditions such as arthritis and TMJ syndrome. If you suffer headaches—even mild ones—do not rely solely on medication. See your primary doctor for diagnosis and care.

Part VII
The Way Things
Ought To Be

In a Perfect World

If he hadn't been so overwhelmed by the momentousness of the occasion, Moses might have been a little disheartened by all those *Thou shalt nots* written on the tablets he carried down from the mountain. "Thou shalt not tell a lie." "Thou shalt not steal." "Thou shalt not kill."

And Moses probably wasn't the most popular guy in the Promised Land, having to tell the Chosen People what they should not do. But the ten commandments had a noble purpose, the establishment of a just and secure society, and without a system of laws this would not have been possible.

Throughout this book, I've had to set forth a series of *don'ts*, a sort of ten commandments of allergy. "Don't use a humidifier." "Don't place a carpet on a cement slab that rests on the ground." "Don't live in a basement apartment."

That's not the way things ought to be. In a perfect world, there wouldn't be any need for me to tell allergic people they should not do these things. Unfortunately, ours isn't a perfect world (if it were, both Moses and I would be out of a job), and allergic people suffer headaches because of humidifiers, carpets, and musty apartments. I must tell them to avoid these things so that they have a chance to live without pain.

But just for a short time, let's put aside the *don'ts* and concentrate on something far more satisfying. Let's pretend you have all the money you need to build a new, perfectly dry home that will forever banish your headache pain. Let's build this dream home in our imagination.

Your finances may not permit building the ideal home, but it won't hurt to fantasize. And perhaps, as we consider the perfect home, it will stimulate some useful ideas for changing your present home, changes that may allow your headaches to subside. If so, describing this imaginary home is worthwhile.

In earlier chapters, we discussed many actions you can take to improve your environment, and this will be a good time to review those recommendations so that you'll be more likely to remember them. It will also reinforce the importance of making these changes to improve your quality of life. Understanding how important it is to correct problems in your home will encourage you to find ways to do so.

Besides, it's fun to imagine a perfect world.

Air Conditioners and Air Cleaners

Before we begin to build our ideal house (or upgrade our present one), we should discuss what measures we will take to improve the quality of the air in the home. For instance, should it have air conditioning and an air cleaner? To answer this question—so frequently asked by my patients—let's look at what these systems can and cannot do.

The Air Conditioner

How delightful it is to leave the oppressive heat and humidity of a blistering hot summer day and enter the sanctuary of a cool, air conditioned house. Soggy with perspiration, we experience such blessed relief as the cool, dry air washes over us.

Besides cooling the home, the air conditioner has another important benefit for the allergic homeowner. It protects against headaches. It does this by drying the air as it cools it, depriving dust mites and mold of the humidity in which they thrive. In drier air, their growth rate is retarded, their numbers shrink, and they lose their power to stimulate head pain.

Air conditioners and dehumidifiers operate on the same principle. Warm air blown over refrigerated coils loses its moisture as water separates from the air and remains on the coils. In the air conditioner, this process cools the air and drives down the humidity. The water extracted from the air then drips off the coils into a pan and drains away. The heat extracted from the house air is routed to an outdoor condenser and released into the atmosphere.

The air emerges from the air conditioner drier and cooler. If the basement shares in the air conditioning, it also dries out, discouraging the growth of mites and mold.

Because the air conditioner dries the basement, many of my patients believe they do not need both an air conditioner and a dehumidifier. They often ask me, "If I have an air conditioner, do I also need an expensive dehumidifier? Can't I save money by relying on the air conditioner to dry the basement?"

Although the idea may seem correct, it really isn't. An air conditioner only dries the air on hot days when the air is being actively cooled. In other words, it only dries air during warm summer weather when the humidity can condense on the cool coils. Running an air conditioner on days when the weather is cooler circulates the air but does not dry it.

This is an important point and well worth repeating. An air conditioner cannot reduce basement humidity during the cool, rainy days of spring and fall because it does not actively cool the air during these seasons. In these seasons, mites and mold will grow in great numbers unless a dehumidifier is operating.

Therefore, to reduce headaches caused by mites and mold, in addition to an air conditioner, buy a dehumidifier. It will keep the basement drier in spring, summer, and fall. I wish every allergy sufferer could have one in their home.

Incidentally, try not to buy a home during the dry seasons of summer or winter. Shop for your new home in the spring or fall, when you have the best chance of telling whether the basement is damp and musty. Too many of my patients suffer unpleasant surprises when their prized new home, purchased during the dry midsummer or winter, turns musty in the spring and fall.

The Air Cleaner

For the allergic person with headaches, what could be more perfect than a machine that cleans the air of the mites, mold, and other allergens it carries? With an air cleaner, can the headache sufferer say good-bye and good riddance to head pain? Can he or she avoid the difficulty and expense of using dehumidifiers, removing carpets, discarding stuffed furniture, and weeding out stored items?

Unfortunately, the answer is no, and to understand why, we must understand how air cleaners work and what they can and cannot do.

Air cleaning machines are designed to remove from the air of our homes the pollen, dust, mold, mites, and other small inhabitants that become airborne. There are two types of machines, and each one cleans the air differently. Those attached to the furnace are called central units, and they filter the air from the entire house as it travels through the furnace. With self-contained or portable models, only the room in which they are located is filtered.

One type of cleaner uses an elaborate filter system to catch and hold the tiny particles of pollen, mite, and mold blown through the filter by a fan. It works well, trapping the mite and mold particles like a window screen catches the cottonwood that floats on the summer air.

The second type of air cleaner, called an electrostatic air cleaner, cleans the air that is drawn through it by zapping the mite, mold, and other dust particles with a charge of electricity. The electricity sticks to the charged particles and attracts them to an oppositely charged plate that plucks them from the air like a magnet attracts powdered iron. The air then exits the machine, cleansed of its load of dust, mites, and mold. This filter also works well.

Whether one type has advantages over the other is a question best left to the air cleaner salesperson or the manufacturers' literature. I don't know which is more effective, but I do know that in the home of the allergic person, either would be a welcome addition. Air cleaners can help relieve headaches, but how well they work depends on a number of factors.

Cheap or Expensive? Whole-House or Portable?

The cost of an air cleaner and the area it cleans are two of the factors that determine its capability. Both cheap and expensive models are available. The more expensive model will usually clean better than the cheap model. Any money saved by buying the cheaper model will often be lost in medical bills that the expensive model could prevent. It is probably unwise to buy a cheap air cleaner. I recommend buying the model that will clean the air best.

Is an air cleaner that is attached to the furnace better than the portable type? The answer to this question is not clear, but I believe each helps the person who suffers headaches. I give my patients the following advice:

- If a home has central heat and air conditioning ducts, a furnace-mounted filter should be purchased if the homeowner can afford it.

- If the home does not have central ductwork, the headache sufferer should purchase a portable model, if possible.

- If a member of the household has severe allergies (i.e., severe asthma or multiple headaches), having both central and room air cleaners may be more helpful than one system alone.

- If the household has only limited funds for health care, they are far better spent on eliminating the causes of allergy (i.e., moisture and shelters for mites and mold in the basement) than on an air cleaner.

- Neither centrally installed nor room air conditioners eliminate the need to correct home moisture problems.

I gathered the above information from patients who have purchased air cleaners and reported how they affected their headaches. In the case of central air cleaners, my patients often have a hard time deciding whether they help, but I believe they do. However, purchasing a central air cleaner is a waste of money if it is installed in a home with excessive moisture—it can't and won't correct the problem. The money used to buy an air cleaner is far better spent drying out the home.

Patients who buy room air cleaners are more certain they help reduce their headaches—many have told me so. Although I don't know if they always help, I believe they are a worthwhile investment for the allergic person with troublesome headaches.

What an Air Cleaner Can and Cannot Clean

I'm sure the divine architect of the human species had a logical reason for handing out favors with one hand and grief with the other, but I don't know why the grief—allergy—has to be so hard to understand and treat?

Perhaps the head architect intended to make treating headaches simple, but a devilish assistant decided to alter the plans, complicating them immensely. That would explain why, although in theory air cleaning should completely eliminate the airborne particles that cause headaches, in reality it does not.

To understand why this is so, try to think of air as a fluid, just like water. (I know; I have trouble with that concept, too.) Now, imagine yourself in a rowboat riding on this fluid, trying to catch a huge fish. As you reel in the fish, you get so excited you lean too far over the side, lose your footing, and tumble into the water, capsizing the boat. Not only do you get soaking wet, you lose the fish and are in danger of losing everything that was in the boat as well.

Quickly, you right the boat, scramble in, and begin to recover your fishing gear. It's easy to retrieve the seat cushions, oars, and your jacket, which are floating nearby. But the fishing rod, tackle box, and portable compact disc player sink before you can get to them. Wet and disgusted, you realize that this miserable experience has taught you a lesson: If an object does not float, it cannot be retrieved.

It's the same with an air cleaner. Its job is to retrieve and filter airborne particles of mite and mold, but it can only capture those particles that float. Some float easily in the air and are readily trapped by the cleaner. Others sink rapidly and do not remain airborne long enough to be captured by the air cleaner.

When viewed through a microscope, particles that float tend to be tiny. They appear to be no bigger than the dot at the end of this sentence. By comparison, the big, luggy particles that sink quickly from the air look as giant as a paragraph. Although both the small and large particles float for a time, only the small ones remain suspended long enough to reach the air cleaner.

Unfortunately, the big mold particles are as important as the smaller particles in causing headaches. Mites and their droppings (which are potent causes of allergy) are also large and do not float well in the air. Because they sink back into the carpet and onto chairs so rapidly, the air cleaner cannot trap them.

But, if they sink so rapidly, aren't they too big to remain in the air long enough for the homeowner to inhale them? No, I'm afraid not. Whenever someone walks across the carpet or sinks into a stuffed chair, the mite and mold particles are released into the air and the headache sufferer inhales them *before they fall back onto the furniture and carpet.*

Since the large particles remain floating in the air such a short time, an air cleaner that is placed directly in the room may trap them better than a centrally located unit. However, neither type of air cleaner will help unless the home is kept as dry as possible. Let's examine why this is so.

The Value of Air Cleaners

The allergic homeowner is often guilty of asking the air cleaner to do a job it cannot do. In this instance, he is like the frugal homeowner who is moving to a new home and decides to save money by not hiring a moving van. Instead, he decides to move all his belongings using the family car.

Backing the car up to the house, he begins filling it with sheets and towels from the linen cabinet, then stuffs in the clothes from all the closets. On top of that he packs all the mattresses and bed frames, followed by the living room sofa and chairs and the dining room set. Then he gets out a ladder and straps the refrigerator, clothes washer, and dryer on top of the pile. Finally, he wedges the lawn mower and snow blower into the trunk.

Delighted at how much money he is saving, he goes to climb into the car—only to discover that it is so full he can't even squeeze into the driver's seat. Even if he could, the load is so heavy it has flattened his tires. As he dejectedly surveys the results of his labors, he realizes he has made a mistake by asking his car to do a job it could not do.

Don't make the same mistake. The air cleaner is a wonderful machine, but don't ask it to do a job it cannot do. There is a tremendous volume of air in your house—and an air cleaner can only clean a small amount at a time. In areas of your house with excess moisture, the carpets and pads continually shed high levels of mite and mold. These levels are increased by stuffed furniture, books, and stored items. The machine can't possibly clean this overloaded air well enough to keep your head from hurting.

Stop overloading it. You must first reduce the moisture and eliminate the shelters that harbor dust mites and mold before the air cleaner can reach its full potential in trapping the airborne particles that provoke your headaches.

The Perfect Home

Unburdened by financial worries (only in our dreams) and determined to live without head pain (that part is true), let's plunge ahead with building the home where we can live free of headaches—the perfect home.

But will I be able to design the perfect home? Before we begin, I should remind you again that I have never designed or built a home. In fact, I consider it a minor miracle if my hammer doesn't bend the nail I'm driving (okay, it's a major miracle). I am not an expert in home design or construction, so if any of the recommendations I make are unrealistic or even impossible, I apologize in advance.

My only qualification for designing a home is the years I have spent trying to think of ways for my patients to correct problems in their homes that cause headaches. How often do I wish they could move to the perfect home, one without the moisture, mold, house dust mites, and other air contaminants that force them to live with pain.

Well, here is our chance to use some of the ideas we have discussed in creating our ideal home. Whether you are considering building a new home or remodeling your present one, I hope some of my suggestions will help you ease your own headaches.

Finding the Perfect Home Site

Our first task is to find a lot on which to construct our home. Finding a suitable lot is critical. Too many of my patients live in homes (or apartments) that should be ideal for people with headaches but aren't because the lots they are built on have too much moisture.

If a house sits on land near a body of water such as a lake or swamp, the land is probably wet. In addition, because the wind picks up moisture as it passes over these wet areas, the air outside the home is also probably damp.

It took me a long time to understand the significance of the moisture content of the air surrounding the home. I learned of its importance while treating patients who lived in apartments. I used to think that occupying an apartment on or above the second floor would ensure freedom from the moisture that is prevalent on the lower floors. It wasn't long until I began realizing that many of my patients suffered deplorable headaches no matter what floor they lived on.

After questioning these patients about where they lived, I learned that most of their apartments were situated in areas that allowed heavy, moist air from the surrounding land to flow toward them. These apartment sites were often in a river valley or on a low area of ground surrounded by hills. The moist air surrounding these apartments caused their headaches.

I still think it is best for my patients to live in an apartment located on the second floor or higher, but only if the building is relatively new, dry, and not situated in a low or wet area that allows moist air to flow into the living space.

This same need for a dry location applies to homes, including the one we are building. Therefore, we will choose a home site on a hill or on a stretch of flat land with no nearby higher ground. Our site will be well removed from lakes, swamps, and other wet areas and will permit good air passage away from our house.

After finding this plot of ground, we will take one other step. We will hire someone to drill a hole to determine the moisture content of the soil and the depth of the water table. Wet soil or a high water table would keep the concrete slab wet and permit excess moisture to enter the home, which, of course, we do not want.

If you prefer to live in an apartment instead of a house, look for a unit on the second or higher floor of a relatively new building that smells dry, has no nearby body of water, contains no indoor pool, and rests on a hill or on a flat area with no surrounding high ground.

Preparing the Basement

If I dared to be unconventional, I would build our home on stilts. This would allow air to circulate below the house, keeping the lowest level dry. There would be no contact with the ground, no wet cement slab, no humid basement. This would mean reduced mite and mold growth and few or no headaches.

This is not typical construction practice in our northern states. I do not know all the disadvantages of building a home on stilts, but there is an obvious one—the winter cold would freeze the exposed water pipes, causing them to crack. They would have to be insulated and perhaps heated to prevent this from happening.

Whatever the disadvantages, this may be a viable option for those exceptionally sensitive patients who react to the moisture arising from even the driest basement. This home would also ensure a dry lower level for homeowners whose space requirements increase in the future. They could convert this area into usable living space with no worry about humidity rising from the floor.

Since I am basically a stick-in-the-mud traditionalist, I probably would not build a house on stilts, but would choose a traditional basement with a concrete slab as its floor. The basement would extend the full length and breadth of the house, and the slab would be laid over a vapor barrier to retard the flow of moisture from the ground to the basement. The outside surface of the basement walls would be insulated to remove any temptation to insulate the inside surface. Insulation applied to the inside of basement walls is likely to harbor moisture and mold.

If, for some reason, a crawl space were absolutely necessary, I would install an efficient vapor barrier in the ceiling of the crawl space to prevent moisture from penetrating the room above it. I would install a second vapor barrier over the floor of the crawl space and vent the area to the outside. This would bring in fresh outside air to flush out the moisture, mold, yeast, and algae that, despite all our precautions, will still be there.

Let's not forget to install an excellent drainage system and landscape the areas surrounding the foundation so that rainwater is carried away from the house. All roof areas should have gutters to ensure that rain and melted snow also drain away from the house.

Last, but not least, our basement would have no partitions. The air would circulate freely, allowing the dehumidifier to reach the entire area above the concrete slab.

The House

Our house would have two stories, and all living spaces would be confined to the two levels above the basement. All bedrooms would be located on the highest floor.

Insulating the house presents a problem. Modern houses are insulated so tightly that unless the windows remain open, the air inside becomes musty and polluted. We would have to install an air infiltration or air exchange system in our house with enough capacity to flush out the moist, polluted air and replace it with fresh outdoor air. What a shame it would be to build the perfect home and forget to let it breathe.

In the northern states, the attic must be insulated well to prevent ice dams that allow water to seep through the roof. Attic vents should be located where they will not allow driving rain or snow to be blown inside where they could cause rotting.

As for the heating plant, either hot water or hot air systems are acceptable. With hot air heating, air conditioning and air cleaning systems can be integrated easily, since all the ducts for these systems are already in place. Central air conditioning and air cleaning are much less expensive when installed during construction than if they are added later. Since we are trying to build a house that is as dry as possible, a central (or portable) humidifier would be inappropriate, and this expense would be avoided.

Our home would be designed so that the garage would be situated beside, behind, or in front of the house, not beneath it. Thus we would avoid having any living space above a garage.

Outfitting the Home

This part is simple. The walls of the basement would be painted with a moisture-proofing compound and left bare so that moisture and mold could not hide behind paneling or drywall. Any water entering the basement would be noticed immediately and the problem dealt with quickly.

The basement floor would be tiled, and carpeting would be limited to washable throw rugs. The furniture used in the basement would be the type with little or no stuffing. Even better, there wouldn't be any furniture or carpeting in the basement to provide shelter for mites and molds.

A washer, dryer (vented to the outside), workbench, and shelves for glass and metal objects would be appropriate here. Items made of paper or fabric would be stored upstairs. From early spring through late fall, a dehumidifier would run continually to dry the basement air.

(Of course, if we built a nonconformist house on stilts, all these basement precautions would be unnecessary.)

Since we have taken steps to ensure a dry basement, there should be very little moisture to affect carpeting, furniture, and other items located in the rest of the house. As long as the carpet and furniture are in good condition, the growth of mites and mold should be kept to a minimum.

There are two situations where the above advice may not be appropriate. First, it applies to people with average sensitivity. Extremely sensitive people plagued by severe allergy may find the lowered mite and mold levels in rooms with bare floors most important in controlling their allergy. Second, it applies to people living in drier areas of the country. People who live in humid areas may find the dust mites and mold growing in upstairs carpeting and furniture a potent cause of continuing headaches. In either of these situations, bare floors and unstuffed furniture would serve the homeowner better.

Adding to a Home

As our families increase in size, we often need more room. Whether for financial reasons or a desire to stay in a familiar neighborhood, we often choose to build onto a house rather than moving to a new one.

Constructing a home addition should be approached with the same caution used in the original home construction. Converting the garage to living space would be inappropriate because it rests on a cement slab. It is also unwise to build over the garage. Converting an attic to living space is acceptable. Adding a room above a crawl space vented to the outside or adding a new living area over an extension of the basement is also acceptable.

Occupying the House

The fumes from the glues used in paneling, carpets, and various other components of a new house will make the first year or two a difficult time for the occupant who suffers headaches. Using construction materials that give off less fumes will help, as will selecting cabinets and shelving made of hardwood instead of particle board or laminates that are glued. It is also a good idea to store carpeting where it can air out before installation.

It is best to move into our new home in the spring. The warm weather permits keeping the windows open much of the time so that the fumes from the new materials can be cleansed by the gentle breezes, a process that continues through summer and fall. By the time winter forces the homeowner to close the windows, much of the odor has dissipated.

Even though exposure to these fumes is regrettable, building the new home is worth it. It will eventually air out, and the dryness we constructed into the home will soothe headaches for years to come.

* * *

If you have the opportunity to build a new house, plan carefully to ensure its dryness. If you cannot afford to build such a house, I hope you will consider implementing some of the ideas we discussed to improve the house you now occupy. You do not have to live with a musty house or with the headaches it breeds.

Is Allergy Treatment Cost-Effective?

Prior to undergoing allergy treatment, the patients I have treated for headaches lived with frequent, often overwhelming pain. I sympathize with their plight and am grateful that my nurses and I have been able to help them. But I am concerned for those with chronic headaches who, for whatever reason, still suffer greatly because they are not receiving the benefits of allergy treatment.

The primary reason they go without this treatment is because allergy is not being considered as a cause of their headaches. And since it is not being considered, it is not being treated.

For this reason, I think it is important that doctors learn about the allergic causes of sinus, migraine, and cluster headaches. I am frequently invited to speak about headaches, and whenever possible, I accept these invitations and do my best to explain the marvelous help my field has to offer patients who live with chronic pain.

My audiences include many physicians who are familiar with allergy and its role in causing headaches, and who are already referring patients with headaches for allergy treatment. But my audiences also include doctors who, despite a growing body of evidence to the contrary, are still resistant to the idea that allergy causes headaches. I know that their resistance is not due to a lack of sympathy for the headache sufferer. Judging from the questions I am frequently asked when I speak to doctors, I think many believe that treatment of headaches with frequent allergy injections is a poor investment of medical resources. The following example is a case in point.

It Costs Too Much

After finishing a lecture recently, I asked if anyone in the audience had questions, and a distinguished-looking doctor raised his hand. When I recognized him, he stood to ask, "Do you mean to say that all patients with headaches need allergy shots?" From the tone of his voice and his posture, I could tell he was irritated.

"No," I replied. "Headaches can be mild and infrequent or severe and frequent. People with mild headaches that occur rarely may need no more treatment than changes in their environment and diet plus a pain reliever, and perhaps an antihistamine or decongestant. People with more frequent and more painful headaches may not find these measures sufficient to relieve their pain. They may need allergy injections."

"But there are millions of people with severe and frequent headaches," he went on. "I realize that environmental control measures and dietary changes do not add to the cost of medical care, but allergy injections do."

"Environmental control measures are costly for the patient," I replied, still not sure where this exchange was leading.

By now, he had become quite agitated and was speaking very loudly. "In these days when the cost of medical care is already too high, treating these patients with allergy injections will only add to this cost," he insisted. "The businesses that employ workers with headaches and the insurance companies that cover the cost of these treatments won't pay this expense. Furthermore, patients won't take the time from their busy schedules to receive them."

I was flustered by this verbal barrage. I am far more comfortable talking to patients one-on-one than speaking in front of a group, and far more comfortable spending hours in front of a word processor than delivering clever retorts. I am afraid I didn't respond very well to his questions. Later, when I had time to think about what he had said, I had to admit that his opinions are probably shared by many others. I decided I should try to address the issues he raised.

Will the Insurance Industry Cover These Costs?

The people who determine policy in the insurance industry are no different from you and me. They only want their subscribers to receive effective medical care at a reasonable cost. If they recognize the benefits of using allergy injections to control chronic headaches, they would have no reason not to cover the cost of this treatment.

Since insurance industry decision makers also understand the concept of cost-benefit analysis, they would be the first to recognize that allergy injections do not necessarily add to the cost of treating patients with frequent and severe headaches. If successful, they can reduce the amount of money that would otherwise be spent on:

- Headache medications,
- Emergency room care,
- Repeating expensive diagnostic tests,
- Frequent doctor visits.

Patients whose headaches are treated successfully need far fewer medications. Since these medications are often expensive, every dose not used represents a cost savings to insurance carriers.

Another area in which allergy treatment can reduce costs is emergency room care. Patients who experience overwhelming headache pain are often forced to go to an emergency room for help. This care is expensive—a single visit can cost more than several months of injection treatment. If allergy treatment prevents these visits, it is far more cost-effective.

A successfully treated patient also has less need for the expensive diagnostic tests used to search for the cause of headaches. I am not criticizing the use of such tests if a physician is worried about a tumor, aneurysm, sinus infection, or any of the other conditions that cause headaches. When the headaches persist in spite of conventional treatments, expensive tests are often repeated in an effort to find the source of the problem. When allergy treatment brings such headaches under control, it is seldom necessary to repeat these tests.

Another area of cost savings is evident in my practice. I usually ask a patient on injection treatment when they last visited their primary doctor, and they often reply, "Not since I started allergy shots." Prior to starting the injections, many of these patients made frequent visits to their doctors for treatment of headaches or the other illness that strike the untreated allergy sufferer.

Not only is there a cost savings because patients make fewer trips to the doctor, when allergy injections control headaches, the visits become more efficient and less costly. The doctor no longer has to worry about chronic headaches in addition to the many other illnesses patients experience. He or she can concentrate on treating arthritis, high blood pressure, or diabetes without simultaneously having to battle chronic headaches.

Along this same vein, I wonder how cost-effective it is for patients to receive psychological counseling while suffering from chronic headaches. Is it possible for either the patient or the counselor to focus on the psyche while the patient is in pain? How often does this lead to treatment failure?

I think the above instances are ample proof that allergy treatment does not mean added cost to health care providers. Instead, it replaces the costs of unnecessary tests, medications, and doctor and emergency room visits while affording the patient welcome pain relief.

Will the Employer Pay for This Treatment?

We have already answered part of this question—allergy treatment is not an added cost but a replacement cost. For employers, refusing to cover the cost of this treatment does not save money. It simply forces them to pay the alternative cost of doctors trying in vain to control allergic headaches without using allergy treatment.

Employing workers with untreated headaches can be expensive for several reasons. One reason is obvious—people with frequent and severe headaches are likely to have a high rate of absenteeism. The employer must hire additional workers to get the work done or risk losing business if orders or deadlines are not met.

The other reason is less obvious. A business whose employees do not provide competent service with a smile will not be around for long. If the clerk who prepares your egg salad sandwich at the deli snarled at you—would you return? If the paper salesman irritably told the print shop owner he was too busy to service his account, would the shop owner continue to buy supplies from the paper company? If the executive vice president of the manufacturing company has a bad day while making a presentation to a major customer, would the manufacturer keep the customer long?

If the reason these employees make such damaging mistakes is that they are nursing a splitting headache, the cost may not be immediately obvious to the employer, but that doesn't mean it won't show up in the long run. It is difficult for an employee with a painful headache to be cheerful and efficient in dealing with customers.

Employers recognize that a healthy employee is a productive one. If they know that effective allergy treatment for chronic headaches is available, they will not refuse to fund this care. To do otherwise would not be a smart business decision.

Will Patients Take Time from Their Busy Days To Receive Allergy Injections?

This issue is the easiest one for me to address. My patients are already taking allergy injections for chronic headaches and are relieved that their days are no longer filled with pain. They do not let inconvenience keep them from receiving this treatment. They live busy lives, and setting aside time to go for an injection is a hardship, but they are willing to accept this inconvenience to avoid continued suffering and irritability.

Besides, after making the necessary changes in their home environment and diet, many patients find they only need injections every two to four weeks. With a single injection conferring weeks of pain relief, this treatment becomes far more convenient.

The Patient with Headaches Must Aggressively Pursue Treatment

Consider a hypothetical patient, Sylvia, who suffers from severe headaches. Her primary doctor examined her and was unable to find a reason for her pain. All tests were normal, and a neurological consultation provided no explanation. Sylvia continued to experience headaches, and feeling frustrated by the lack of answers, decided to come up with her own answers:

- "I must have tension headaches."

- "They must come from trouble in my marriage (or work, or school)."

- "I must be overreacting to this pain."

Sylvia's answers imply that her discomfort arises from an inability to respond to the tensions and anxieties in her life. Is this true? Should she resign herself to living with her headaches and stop searching for other possibilities?

I would encourage Sylvia to continue searching for answers. While there is no doubt that anxiety and tension exert a powerful influence in some cases of chronic headaches, in many other cases, they play only a minor role. Even in people who are strongly affected by anxiety and tension, I wonder whether these debilitating feelings represent the entire cause, or only part of the cause. If they are only part of the cause, then other treatments, including those of allergy, have an excellent chance of helping to relieve their pain.

If medical conditions other than tension and anxiety are diagnosed and treated, and if frequent and painful headaches persist in spite of this treatment, continuing to search for additional causes of pain is certainly appropriate.

* * *

Become a knowledgeable medical consumer. Tell your doctor that you want to know why you have headaches and you want to learn how to treat them.

See a neurologist, dentist, psychologist, or any other specialist who might help you. Agree to have any pertinent tests. Use any recommended medication. Aggressively pursue the cause of your headaches, and do not accept anything less than the best treatment available.

If your headaches persist, return to your primary doctor. Explain that you continue to have pain, and ask where to go next. That's how many of my patients finally found their way to my office.

Many people suffer allergic headaches that could be treated. I hope this book will help teach them about the relief allergy treatment provides. Many doctors could provide this relief. I hope this book will help teach them how to provide this relief. If it does, I will be most pleased.

Bibliography

Arlian, L. G.; Bernstein, D.; Bernstein, I. L.; Friedman, S.; Grant, A.; Leiberman, P.; Lopez, M., Metzger, J.; Platts-Mills, T.; Schatz, M.; Spector, S.; Wasserman, S. I.; Zeiger, R. S. "Prevalence of Dust Mites in the Homes of People Living in Eight Different Geographic Areas of the United States," *The Journal of Allergy and Clinical Immunology*, Vol. 90, No. 3, Pt. 1, September 1992: pp. 292–300.

Burnet, C.; Bedard, P. M.; Lavoie, A.; Jobin, M.; Hebert, J. "Allergic Rhinitis to Ragween Pollen. I. Reassessment of the Effects of Immunotherapy on Cellular and Humoral Responses," *The Journal of Allergy and Clinical Immunology*, Vol. 89, No. 1, Pt. 1, January 1992: pp. 76–86.

Burnet, C.; Bedard, P. M.; Lavoie, A.; Jobin, M.; Hebert, J. "Allergic Rhinitis to Ragween Pollen. II. Modulation of Histamine-Releasing Factor Production by Specific Immunotherapy," *The Journal of Allergy and Clinical Immunology*, Vol. 89, No. 1, Pt. 1, January 1992: pp. 87–94.

Claman, H. N. "The Biology of the Immune Response," *The Journal of the American Medical Association*, Vol. 269, No. 20, November 25, 1992: pp. 2790–6.

Consumers Union reprint. "The Shot Doctors," *Consumers Report*, February 1988, pp. 1–4.

Creticos, P. S. "Immunotherapy with Allergens," *The Journal of the American Medical Association*, Vol. 269, No. 20, November 25, 1992: pp. 2834–39.

Dales, R.; Burnett, R.; and Zwanenburg, H. "Adverse Health Effects Among Adults Exposed to Home Dampness and Mold," *American Review of Respiratory Disease*, Vol. 143, No. 3, March 1991: pp. 505–9.

de Boer, R. "The Control of House Dust Mite Allergens in Rugs," *The Journal of Allergy and Clinical Immunology*, Vol. 86, No. 5, November 1990: pp. 808–14.

Dhillin, M. "Current Status of Mold Immunotherapy," *The Annals of Allergy*, Vol. 66, No. 5, May 1991: pp. 385–92.

Diamond, S. (ed.) "Headaches," *The Medical Clinics of North America*, 75(3), May 1991, pp. 521–789.

Dietemann, A.; Bessot, J.; Hoyet, C.; Ott, Verot A.; Pauli, G. "A Double Blind, Placebo Controlled Trial of Solidified Benzyl Benzoate Applied in the Dwellings of Asthmatic Patients Sensitive to Mites: Clinical Efficacy and Effect on Mite Allergens," *The Journal of Allergy and Clinical Immunology*, Vol. 91, No.3, March 1993: pp. 738–46.

Evans, R. "Environmental Control and Immunotherapy for Allergic Disease," *The Journal of Allergy and Clinical Immunology*, Vol. 90, No. 3, Pt. 2, September 1992: pp. 462–8.

Frew, A. J.; and O'Hehir, R. E. "What Can We Learn From Studies of Lymphocytes Present in Allergic Reaction Sites?" *The Journal of Allergy and Clinical Immunology*, Vol. 89, No. 4, April 1992: pp. 783–8.

Hudzinski, L. G.; and Frohlich, E. D. "One-Year Longitudinal Study of a No-Smoking Policy in a Medical Institution," *Chest*, Vol. 97, No. 5, May 1990: pp. 1198–1202; Comment in: *Chest*, pp. 1027–8.

Karlsson-Borga, A.; Jonssom, P.; and Rolfson, W. "Specific IgE Antibodies to 16 Widespread Mold Genera in Patients with Suspected Mold Allergy," *The Annals of Allergy*, Vol. 63, No. 6, Pt. 1, December 1989: pp. 521–6.

Levi, R.; Edman, G. V.; Ekbom, K.; and Waldenlind, E. "Episodic Cluster Headache. II: High Tobacco and Alcohol Consumption in Males," *Headache*, Vol. 32, No. 4, April 1992: pp. 184–7.

Lyles, W. B. "Sick Building Syndrome," *The Southern Medical Journal*, Vol. 84, No. 1, January 1991: pp. 65–71.

McDonald, L. G.; and Tovey, E. "The Role of Water Temperature and Laundry Procedures in Reducing House Dust Mite Populations and Allergen Content of Bedding," *The Journal of Allergy and Clinical Immunology*, Vol. 90, No. 4, Part 1, October 1992.

Middleton, M.; Reed, C. E.; Ellis, E. F.; Adkinson, N. F.; Yunginger, J. W.; and Busse, W. W. *Allergy, Principles and Practice*. St. Louis: Mosby, 1993.

Mondell, B. E. "Evaluation of the Patient Presenting With Headache," *The Medical Clinics of North America*, Vol. 75, No. 3, May 1991: pp. 521–4.

Nordvall, S. L.; Agrell, B.; Malling, H. J.; and Dreborg, S. "Diagnosis of Mold Allergy by RAST and Skin Prick Testing," *The Annals of Allergy*, Vol. 65, No. 5, November 1990: pp. 418–22.

O'Hallaren, M. T.; Yunginger, J. W.; Offord, K. P.; Somers, M. J.; O'Connell, E. J.; and Ballard, D. J. "Exposure to an Aeroallergen as a Possible Precipitating Factor in Respiratory Arrest in Young Patients with Asthma," Comment in: *The New England Journal of Medicine*, Vol. 34, No. 6, February 7, 1991: pp. 409–11.

Olesen, J. "The Classification and Diagnosis of Headache Disorders," *The Neurological Clinics* (United States), Vol. 8, No. 4, November 1990: pp. 793–9.

Oppenheimer, J. J.; Nelson, H. S.; Bock, S. A.; Christensen, F.; and Leung, D. Y. M. "Treatment of Peanut Allergy with Rush Immunotherapy," *The Journal of Allergy and Clinical Immunology*, Vol. 90, No. 2, August 1992: pp. 256–9.

Payne, T. J.; Stetson, B.; Stevens, V. M.; Johnson, C. A.; Penzien, D. B.; and Van Dorsten, B. "The Impact of

Cigarette Smoking on Headache Activity in Headache Patients," *Headache,* Vol. 31, No. 5, May 1991: pp. 329–32.

Platt, S. D.; Martin, C. J.; Hunt, S. M.; and Lewis, C. W. "Damp Housing, Mould Growth, and Symptomatic Health State," *British Medical Journal,* Vol. 298, No. 6689, July 29, 1989: p. 1673–8.

Pollart, S.; Chapman, M. D.; and Platts-Mills, T. A. E. *Clinical Reviews in Allergy,* Vol. 6, 1988: pp. 23–33.

Reisman, R. E.; Mauriello, P. M.; Davis, G. B.; Georgitis, J. W.; and DeMasi, J. M. "A Double Blind Study of the Effectiveness of a High-Effeciency Particulate Air (HEPA) Filter in the Treatment of Patients with Perennial Allergic Rhinitis," *The Journal of Allergy and Clinical Immunology,* Vol. 85, No. 6, June 1990, pp. 1050–7.

Rieckenberg, M. R.; Khan, R. H.; and Day, J. H. "Physician Reported Patient Response to Immunotherapy: A Retrospective Study of Factors Affecting the Response," *The Annals of Allergy,* Vol. 64, No. 4, April 1990: pp. 364–7.

Saper, J. R. "Daily Chronic Headache," *The Neurological Clinics* (United States), Vol. 8, No. 4, November, 1990: pp. 891–901.

Schwartz, J.; and Zeger, S. "Passive Smoking, Air Pollution, and Acute Respiratory Symptoms in a Diary Study of Student Nurses," *American Review of Respiratory Diseases,* Vol. 141, No. 1, January 1990: pp. 62–7.

Seidenari, S.; Manzini, B. M.; Danese, P; and Giannetti, A. "Positive Patch Tests to Whole Mite Cultures and Purified Mite Extracts in Patients with Atopic Dermatitis, Asthma, and Rhinitis," *The Annals of Allergy,* Vol. 69, September, 1992: pp. 201–6.

Sprenger, J. D.; Altman, L. C.; O'Neil, C. E.; Ayars, G. H.; Butcher, B. T.; and Lerher, S. B. "Prevalence of Basidiospore Allergy in the Pacific Northwest," *The Journal of Allergy and Clinical Immunology,* Vol. 82, No. 6, December 1988: pp. 1076–80.

Stewart, G. E.; and Lockey, R. F. "Systemic Reactions from Allergen Immunotherapy," Editorial in: *The Journal of Allergy and Clinical Immunology*, Vol. 90, No. 4, Pt. 1, October 1992: pp. 567–78.

Swanson, M. C.; Campbell, A. R.; Klauck, M. J.; and Reed, C. E. "Correlations Between Levels of Mite and Cat in Settled and Airborne Dust," *The Journal of Allergy and Clinical Immunology*, Vol. 83, No. 4, April 1989: pp. 776–83.

Wickman, M.; Gravesen, S.; Nordvall, S.; Pershagen, G.; and Sundell, J. "Indoor Viable Dust-bound Microfungi in Relation to Residential Characteristics, Living Habits, and Symptoms in Atopic and Control Children," *The Journal of Allergy and Clinical Immunology*, Vol. 89, No. 3, March 1992: pp. 752–9.

Wood, R. A.; Eggleston, P. A.; Lind, P.; Ingeman, L.; Schwartz, B.; Graveson, S.; Terry, D.; Wheeler, B.; and Adkinson, N. F. "Antigenic Analysis of Household Dust Samples," *American Review of Respiratory Disease*, Vol. 37, No. 2, February 1988: pp. 358–63.

Yoshida, K.; Ando, M.; Sakata, T.; and Araki, S. "Environmental Mycological Studies on the Causative Agent of Summer Type Hypersensitivity Pneumonitis," *The Journal of Allergy and Clinical Immunology*, Vol. 81, No. 2, February 1988: pp. 475–83.